BREATHING EASY

BREATHING EASY

A HANDBOOK FOR ASTHMATICS

The Acclaimed Treatment Program from the
National Jewish Center for Immunology
and Respiratory Medicine

Genell Subak-Sharpe

James V. Warren, M.D.,
Consulting Editor

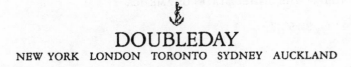

DOUBLEDAY
NEW YORK   LONDON   TORONTO   SYDNEY   AUCKLAND

Published by DOUBLEDAY, a division of Bantam Doubleday Dell Publishing Group, Inc., 666 Fifth Avenue, New York, New York 10103.

DOUBLEDAY and the portrayal of an anchor with a dolphin are trademarks of Doubleday, a division of Bantam Doubleday Dell Publishing Group, Inc.

NOTE TO THE READER

The ideas, procedures, and suggestions in this book are not intended as a substitute for consultation with your physician. For the proper diagnosis and treatment of asthma, a doctor's supervision is suggested.

All drawings are courtesy of The National Jewish Center for Immunology and Respiratory Medicine.

Library of Congress Cataloging-in-Publication Data
Subak-Sharpe, Genell J.
    Breathing easy.

    (The Frontiers of medicine series)
    Includes index.
    1. Asthma—Popular works. I. Warren, James V.
(James Vaughn), 1915– . II. National Jewish Center
for Immunology and Respiratory Medicine (U.S.) III. Title.
IV. Series. [DNLM: 1. Asthma—popular works. WF 553 S941b]
RC591.S78 1988   616.2'38   87-15726

ISBN 0-385-23440-6
Copyright © 1988 by G.S. Sharpe Communications, Inc.
ALL RIGHTS RESERVED
PRINTED IN THE UNITED STATES OF AMERICA

2 4 6 8 9 7 5 3

BG

ACKNOWLEDGMENTS

The creation of any book inevitably represents the efforts of many people, and this is particularly true in this instance. Dozens of dedicated physicians, nurses, psychologists, therapists, and other staff members at the National Jewish Center for Immunology and Respiratory Medicine have devoted many hours to this project. They have shared the understanding and knowledge gained through years of patient care and have provided us with materials they have prepared for patients at the National Jewish Center. Thanks to their unstinting cooperation, we can truly say that this book reflects the multifaceted approach to asthma that has made National Jewish the premier institution in its field.

Unfortunately, space does not permit naming all the people who have contributed to this book. Some, however, deserve special mention. Dr. Robert Mason has kept us on course throughout the project, giving us free run of the hospital, enlisting members of his staff for interviews, providing vital background material, checking our facts, and, most importantly, sharing his special insight. Other National Jewish staff members who have been particularly helpful include Drs. Dan Atkins, Bruce Bender, Robert A. Bethel, Manon Brenner, Reuben M. Cherniack, Philip Corsello, Richard Farr, Enrique Fernandez, Charles Irvin, Michael G. Moran, David A. Mrazek, Bruce D. Miller, Richard Strunk, and Stanley Szefler. Nurses Laura Neilley and Rosemary Simpkins provided special insight into what goes on in the various patient wards; Susan Ludwick showed us what is involved in exercise conditioning and rehabilitation. The patients we interviewed, whose names and histories have been disguised in this book, told us what it really means to have asthma. To each of them we extend special thanks for being so open and so sharing.

Jane Margaretten-Ohring has spent long hours poring through reference books to compile accurate and meaningful tables on tests and drugs. Finally, I want to thank my husband, Gerald, and my children David, Sarah, and Hope for their patience and for pitching in when needed.

CONTENTS

CONTENTS

FOREWORD

Asthma is a common chronic illness that affects about 7 percent of the adult population sometime during their lives, with asthma symptoms occuring in about 3 percent of adults in current cross-sectional national surveys. What makes asthma so difficult is its variability. The disease can be very mild or devastating, can first occur in infancy or in the elderly, and can be much more severe at different times in one's life. We all wish we could cure asthma, but we cannot. We can, however, treat the symptoms of asthma and bring the disease under control. The symptoms of asthma may disappear for years or decades, but they are likely to recur. Asthma is essentially hyperreactive airways or "twitchy lungs;" once the airways are irritable, many nonspecific irritants can trigger asthmatic attacks. The triggering factors may be allergies, a host of nonspecific irritants, and a variety of nonimmunologic factors. Therapy has two goals. One is to relieve symptoms and the other is to reduce the underlying airway reactivity. (Specific treatments are discussed throughout this book.) Sometimes it is difficult for patients to realize that they may need intensive therapy for several months to allow the irritable airways to heal so that they are not so hyperreactive and twitchy. Once the airways have recovered or healed, less medicine is required and nonspecific irritants are less troublesome.

Asthma can be very scary. There are few human experiences as frightening as being short of breath or suffocating. This feeling is compounded if one doesn't know when it will occur or how severe it will be. Most asthma is mild and easily controlled medically. However, chronic asthma can be devastating. The disease can cause respiratory impairment and disability. Oral corticosteroids such as prednisone, which must be used to control severe asthma, may produce changes in physical appearance such as obesity and a rounded face, as well as internal changes such as thinning bones and muscle weakness. The net result of the combination of severe disease and a medical regimen with significant side effects can be depression, anxiety, anger, and withdrawal from society. The purpose of this book is to prevent this tragic outcome, which unfortunately we see every day.

The key to the medical management of any chronic disease is patient education. Without patient education, no therapy will work. Surgeons are fortunate, for there are some diseases that can be cured with a scalpel. However, medical diseases like asthma require patients' cooperation and participation in their therapy. For most diseases, the best treatment is prevention. The prevention of worsening asthma is to educate the patient about the disease, the treatment, the anticipated psychosocial issues of having a chronic disease, and the use of a peak flow meter to monitor the disease at home. The purpose of this book is to provide part of that education. The rest of the education should come from your physician, nurses, and therapists.

National Jewish Center for Immunology and Respiratory Medicine is the "National Asthma Center." From 1978 to 1985, the official name of National Jewish was National Jewish Hospital/National Asthma Center. The change in the name in 1985 was to reflect the long-term research programs in basic immunology and other clinical respiratory diseases such as emphysema, pulmonary fibrosis, sleep disorders, and drug-resistant tuberculosis. Each year we see patients from nearly all fifty states and about ten foreign countries. Most people come as outpatients, but those with severe disease are treated as impatients. Most patients come because their disease cannot be controlled at home or to get a second opinion. From my perspective, one of the major reasons for coming should be for patient education, which is the focus of this book. To care for asthma, one must understand the disease and the medical treatment program.

In its early days, National Jewish was supported almost entirely by contributions. It proudly proclaimed that it took only those patients who could not pay for their care. Even today, patients are charged on the basis of what they can pay. Research grants and contributions still provide about half of our operating revenue.

Scientists at National Jewish cover a broad spectrum of research ranging from basic molecular and cellular biology to clinical testing of new drugs. Many of the world's authorities in immunology are here, carrying on research, into this still largely unknown area, that is instrumental in virtually all aspects of medicine. It is our hope that our basic science will ultimately lead to better therapy for asthma as well as other respiratory and immunologic diseases.

The focus of this book is on rehabilitation. At National Jewish, rehabilitation is synonymous with treatment. At first, many of our patients feel they have no need for rehabilitation —they think that rehabilitation is intended for people with physical handicaps. In our view, rehabilitation means achieving your full potential—reducing the number of sick days from school or work, being able to participate fully in family and community activities, leading a more active life without the constant fear of a frightening attack of not being able to breathe. It also means facing the often paralyzing anger that prevents many people with a chronic disease from maintaining satisfactory relationships. Our approaches to these varied aspects of living with asthma are described in this book.

Even if asthma cannot be cured, it can be controlled, and nearly all asthmatics can lead a normal life. The key is to know what triggers one's asthma, how to prevent and treat attacks, and how to deal with the knowledge of having a chronic disease. We hope that this book will be useful to patients with asthma. Our approach is based on established scientific and medical practice. We do not have a secret cure.

Our success is related to our comprehensive program and our ability to develop specific treatment programs for individual patients. Our goal is to develop individualized treatment programs so as to maximize one's daily activity while at the same time using the minimal amount of medicines necessary to achieve and to sustain the maximal function. We try to develop a program that places the fewest restrictions on daily life and encourages maximal activity, including a daily exercise program. Each asthmatic is different, and each needs an individualized treatment program. Although as a physician I would like to attribute our success to the expertise and dedication of our doctors, the truth is that the real cause for success is the dedication and personal involvement of our nurses, therapists, psychologists, educators, and other health professionals. They have extensive experience dealing with patients with chronic respiratory and immunologic diseases.

This book presents our basic multifaceted approach to asthma. At National Jewish, we feel that it is vital for patients and family members to learn as much as possible about their disease and approaches to treatment. A patient who truly understands what is happening has a head start in gaining control over his or her disease and leading a normal life. Of course, a book is not intended to enable you to become an informed partner in your own medical care. From this book, you will learn how the lungs function normally and what happens during an attack of asthma. You will learn how we go about identifying factors that worsen asthma and what you can do to eliminate or minimize them. You also will learn how to get the most out of asthma treatments, especially the inhaled treatments.

To help answer questions about respiratory and immunologic diseases, we have established the LUNG Line (1-800-222-LUNG). This toll-free telephone information service has been in existence for four years. Questions are answered by specially trained nurses and by other National Jewish staff members as appropriate.

The creation of this book is in keeping with our basic goal of providing authoritative and practical information about asthma. It contains many of the charts and materials we have prepared for our patients. Readers should not use this information to alter their own treatment regimen without checking with their doctors. If you think the approaches described on the following pages might be useful for you or a family member, show this book to your doctor.

Robert J. Mason, M.D.
Chairman, Department of Medicine
National Jewish Center for
Immunology and Respiratory Medicine
Denver, Colorado

CHAPTER 1

Your Lungs and How They Work

In order to understand—and control—asthma, it is important to first understand how lungs normally function. Actually, breathing is something that most of us take for granted. Without conscious thought or effort, each one of us takes an average of 10 to 15 breaths per minute, day in and day out, from the moment of birth onwards. The average adult takes in more than 12,000 quarts of air a day. We take in more air than any other substance, and we can live for only a few minutes without it.

With luck and care, lungs will last a lifetime, but along the way there are scores of factors that can cause breathing difficulties. This book focuses on one of the more common diseases: asthma—or to use the technical name, *reversible obstructive airway disease.*

The Respiratory System

The human respiratory system is marvelously engineered with millions of parts working together to provide clean, filtered oxygen from the air to the circulatory system and to remove carbon dioxide, a gaseous waste product, from the body. (Figure 1 shows the major parts of the respiratory system.) Each time you breathe, air is inhaled through the nostrils or mouth. As the air travels to the throat, it passes through the nose and then the adenoids and tonsils, which begin the process of filtering out harmful substances such as bacteria or other disease-causing organisms. The nose and other structures in the upper airway also warm and moisten the air. For a short distance, air and food travel along the same passageway in the throat; but just at the top of the *larynx,* or voice box, air passes through the *glottis,* which is protected by the *epiglottis,* a kind of trapdoor that allows the passage of air, but closes to keep water or food out of the *trachea,* or windpipe. Sometimes the epiglottis may close improperly or not soon enough to prevent the passage of a small amount of food or water into the larynx. This results in the choking characteristically referred to as "going down the wrong pipe." Normally, however, it is impossible to breath and swallow at the same time. Since air is needed for proper speech, when we exhale it passes through the larynx on its way from the lungs to the mouth.

The airways can be likened to an inverted tree, with the trachea as the trunk; the left and right bronchi as the two main branches; the bronchioles as increasingly smaller branches and twigs; and the *alveoli,* the tiny bubble-like air sacs, as the leaves (see Figure 2). On its journey through the pulmonary tree, the air is warmed to body temperature. It is also filtered, purified, and moistened. Microscopic, hairlike structures called *cilia* as well as millions of tiny mucus-producing glands line the air passages (see Figure 3). The sticky mucus filters out and traps impurities that may be in the air; it also moistens the air so that it will not dry out the lungs. The cilia move in a coordinated, wavelike motion to keep the mucus moving and fresh. As the cilia move the mucus from the lower part of the lungs to the top of the pulmonary tree, the impurities are carried along with it; they are eventually deposited either in the nasal passages where they can be sneezed out of the body, or in the throat where they are

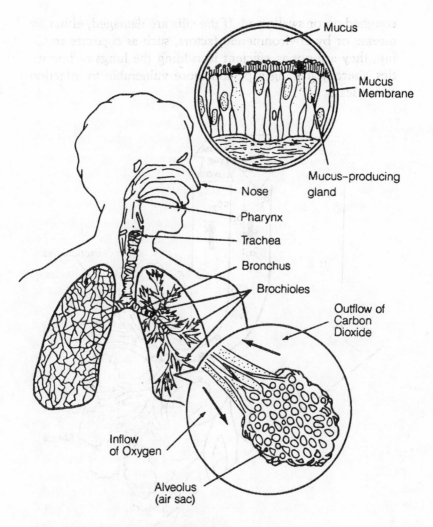

Mucus

Mucus Membrane

Mucus-producing gland

Nose

Pharynx

Trachea

Bronchus

Brochioles

Outflow of Carbon Dioxide

Inflow of Oxygen

Alveolus (air sac)

Figure 1
NORMAL LUNG ANATOMY

coughed up or swallowed. If the cilia are damaged, either by disease or by environmental factors, such as cigarette smoking, they are not as efficient in ridding the lungs of impurities, thereby making a person more vulnerable to infection and disease.

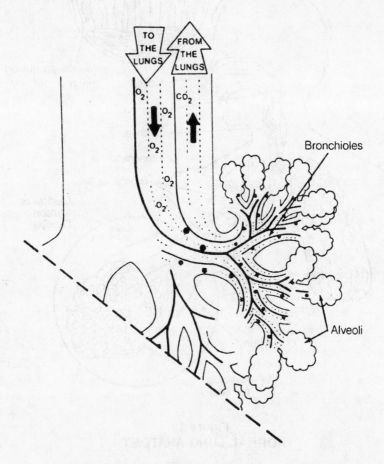

Figure 2
ENLARGEMENT OF NORMAL AIRWAY
Note the branching into smaller and smaller airways as they go deeper into the lung and end in tiny air sacs, each of which is called an alveolus.

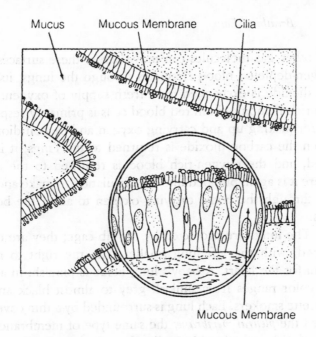

Figure 3
ENLARGEMENT OF NORMAL MUCOUS MEMBRANE

The average lung contains 300 to 400 million alveoli. When viewed under a microscope, these tiny sacs look like clusters of grapes. It is in these microscopic sacs that the true process of respiration—the exchange of blood gases—takes place.

Every body cell requires oxygen to live. About 20 percent of the air we breathe in is made up of oxygen; most of the rest is nitrogen, with tiny amounts of other gases. Just as a fire needs oxygen in order to burn its fuel, so, too, does the body require oxygen to convert its fuel, which is derived from food, into energy. Although the lungs are located within the chest cavity, the inner surfaces of the alveoli and the air passages are actually exposed to the outside environment. The inner surfaces of the alveoli are in contact with capillaries, the tiniest of blood vessels. The walls of both the capillaries and alveoli are only one cell thick; thus oxygen and other gas molecules can move across these surfaces. As oxygen-depleted blood circulates through the lungs, its carbon dioxide is exchanged for a fresh supply of oxygen. The iron-rich hemoglobin in red blood cells is primarily responsible for picking up and carrying oxygen and carbon dioxide. When the carbon dioxide is returned to the lungs, it is exhaled, and the oxygen-rich blood is returned to the heart where it is again pumped into the circulation to make another trip through the body, carrying oxygen to all of the body's cells.

The lungs are protected by the rib cage; they are cone-shaped, with the left lung smaller than the right to make room for the heart. A baby's lung tissue is pinkish; in adults the color ranges from pinkish grey to almost black among cigarette smokers. Each lung is surrounded by a thin covering called the *pleural membrane;* the same type of membrane also lines the chest cavity. Normally, there is almost no space between the two membranes, which are lubricated by a fluid so that they can glide easily over each other as the lungs expand and contract with each breath. Sometimes, however, the linings may become inflamed and rub against each other, resulting in a painful condition called *pleurisy.*

How We Breathe

At the moment of birth, a baby's lungs contain no air, and appear to be solid masses. During gestation the fetal lungs are filled with fluid, most of which is squeezed out through the mouth during birth; the little that remains is absorbed by the baby's body. With a baby's first breath, the lungs expand to fill the space available within the chest cavity. Lung tissue is very elastic, and the lungs are kept expanded by the pull of negative pressure, or vacuum, of the pleural cavity that encases them. A lung may collapse if there is a break in this vacuum, which acts like an air seal. For example, if air from inside the lung escapes into the pleural cavity through a ruptured alveolus, it can result in a collapsed lung. Similarly, an injury that allows outside air to enter the pleural cavity can collapse a lung.

Movement of the ribs and the *diaphragm*—the major muscle used for respiration—is responsible for the expansion and contraction of the lungs, forcing the air in and out; this is similar to what happens when a bellows is worked. The breathing muscles of the chest and the rate at which we breathe are regulated by a center of nerves in the *medulla*, a structure of the lower brain located at the top of the spinal cord.

Breathing is mostly automatic, but it can also be a voluntary action. When a doctor tells you to take a deep breath and hold it, for example, you can consciously follow those instructions. Most of the time, however, we breathe automatically and without thinking about it. The rate at which we breathe is controlled by a delicate feedback system. When oxygen drops to a certain level, or a certain amount of carbon dioxide builds up in the blood, a message is sent to the medulla directing the person to inhale. You can test this feedback system yourself by attempting to hold your breath. After a minute or so, the urge to inhale becomes so overpowering that you can no longer resist it. Sometimes a child will hold his or her breath in an attempt to gain attention, and succeed until he or she turns blue in the face. The youngster may even fall to the floor in a faint but will automatically start breathing. Indeed, it is impossible to commit suicide by holding your breath; you may be able to make yourself faint, but then you will resume breathing even against your will.

The lungs are capable of taking in much more air than is needed to perform ordinary functions. This is fortunate; a person can lose an entire lung and still not experience shortness of breath. In a normal breath, about a pint of air flows in and out of the lungs. This is only about an eighth of our total lung capacity. If a person with healthy lungs continues inhaling beyond a normal breath, five to six extra pints of air may be taken in. Similarly, a person with healthy lungs can force out an extra pint and a half of supplemental air. But it is impossible to completely empty the lungs; about a pint and a half of residual air will remain in the average adult's lungs no matter how forcefully he or she exhales. Even a lung that has collapsed after being removed from the body will retain enough air to float in water. An exception is the lung of a stillborn infant—in fact, doubts as to whether or not the baby was dead at birth can be resolved by determining whether the lungs sink or float. If they sink, it is proof that the baby did not breathe and was stillborn.

Other Functions of the Lungs

Although maintaining a steady supply of oxygen is the lungs' most vital function, they have other important roles. For example, the lungs are one of our major protectors against airborne microorganisms, pollutants, and other potentially harmful substances. Even though the lungs are classified as internal organs, vast amounts of their inner surface actually are exposed to the outside environment. Typically, we think that the skin has the largest exposed surface of any vital organ; in reality, however, its total surface in an adult is about two square yards, compared to a total "exposed" surface equal to that of a tennis court for the lungs.

The lungs have several protective mechanisms that prevent harmful substances from entering the body. For example, the tiny airways are encircled by bands of smooth-muscle tissue. When a person breathes in potentially harmful particles, such as dust or asbestos fibers, these muscles automatically constrict and limit the flow of air into the lungs. Most dusts or particles are removed by the concerted sweeping action of the cilia. But despite such highly efficient protective systems, some harmful substances inevitably escape and enter the lungs and bloodstream. Still, the healthier the lungs, the more protection they offer against airborne diseases and hazards.

The lungs also serve as processors of many of the chemicals carried to them via the blood. For example, a body chemical instrumental in maintaining blood pressure, *angiotensin II,* is formed in the lungs. Similarly, the capillaries in the lung can also inactivate chemicals that alter blood pressure. A number of other important metabolic functions, many of which are not fully understood, are also carried out in the lungs.

CHAPTER 2

What Is Asthma?

Asthma is a chronic disease that afflicts between nine and ten million Americans. It is a complex disease that has baffled and challenged physicians for centuries. Although the disease may make itself evident in a variety of ways, all asthma patients from time to time have difficulty breathing. The problem is caused by very sensitive, or hyperreactive, airways that constrict or narrow, cutting down on the flow of air in and out of the lungs. Doctors at the National Jewish Center often describe the condition as "twitchy lungs." Patients often say an asthma attack is "like breathing through a straw," and that it leaves them hungry for air.

Several things happen during an asthma attack to produce the characteristic feeling of air hunger. The tiny muscles that encircle the bronchial tubes go into spasm—the medical term for what is happening is "bronchospasm"—causing the airways to narrow and cut off some of the flow of air. (See Figures 4 and 5.) A similar but less intense tightening of the bronchial muscles occur in people who do not have asthma when they are exposed to large amounts of smoke, noxious fumes, or other pollutants. This is one way that the body attempts to protect itself against the invasion of potentially

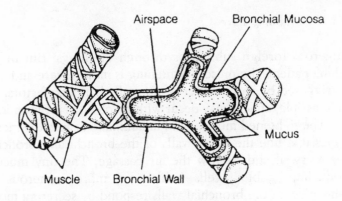

Figure 4
NORMAL BRONCHIOLE

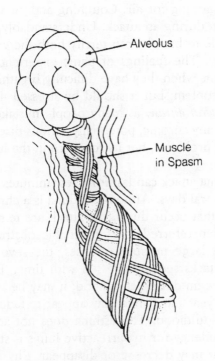

Figure 5
BRONCHOSPASM

dangerous foreign substances through the lungs. But in an asthma patient, the muscle tightening is more severe and can be triggered by any number of normally harmless factors. In some people, attacks may occur with no obvious provocation.

The tightened muscles and inflammation cause the membranes that line the inner walls of the bronchi and bronchioles to swell and narrow the air passage. The tiny mucus-producing "goblet" cells (which are more numerous in asthmatics) in the bronchial walls respond by secreting more mucus. This mucus builds up in the bronchial tubes, further clogging the tiny air passages and blocking air flow (see Figure 6). Stale air becomes trapped in the alveoli, causing a buildup of carbon dioxide and resulting in breathlessness, or a feeling of gasping for air. Coughing and/or wheezing are very common during an attack. Understandably, a feeling of not being able to breathe can terrify both the victim and his or her family. The feelings of panic experienced by many asthma patients when they have difficulty breathing can exacerbate the problem; but it should be stressed that asthma *is not a psychological disease,* as many people mistakenly assume. Asthma, like any chronic, potentially serious disease, can lead to emotional problems, but its roots are in the lungs, not the head.

An asthma attack can last for a few minutes or, in severe cases, for several days. Although asthma is a chronic disease, the changes that occur during an attack are temporary; thus asthma is often referred to as reversible obstructive airway disease. In a large number of cases, the severity and frequency of attacks seems to lessen with time. Typically, the asthma will begin during childhood; it may be severe during the growing years, and then may appear to fade during adolescence or adulthood. The asthma does not actually disappear—the tendency for hyperreactive lungs is still there, but the symptoms may decrease or disappear. Physicians do not know why this happens, but many believe that it is related to the natural growth and development of the lungs. The effects

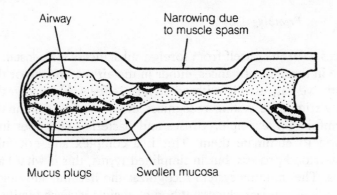

Figure 6
BLOCKED AIRWAY

Airway

Narrowing due to muscle spasm

Mucus plugs

Swollen mucosa

of asthma are more pronounced in the smaller bronchioles. As a child grows, the proportion of very small bronchioles decreases as the larger airways develop, so the airflow is not impeded as much. Not uncommonly, the asthma may reappear later, but often in a milder form than during its early years. There are, however, exceptions. Sometimes the disease worsens during adolescence, and may even lead to death. In other instances, it may first appear during adulthood and become progressively severe with age. Fortunately, severe progressive asthma is relatively rare; although asthma can be a disruptive disease, with proper care the large majority of patients can lead normal, productive lives.

Causes of Asthma

The fundamental cause of asthma is unknown, but its effects and triggering factors are well understood. In perhaps as many as two out of three children and one out of three adults with asthma, the attacks are related to an immune response to specific environmental factors. These patients often have a history of allergies and will develop hives during skin tests with specific allergens. Blood tests may show high levels of immunoglobulin E, or IgE, an antibody that the body produces to protect itself from foreign substances. We constantly take in foreign substances, either in the air we breathe or the foods we eat, usually with no adverse effects. Normally, the body's immune system recognizes those that are potentially harmful—for example, viruses and bacteria—and goes into action to eliminate them. This is a complex and not fully understood process, but in simplified terms, this is what happens. The immune system recognizes the harmful substance, or antigen, and produces antibodies against it. Each family of antibodies is programmed to recognize a specific antigen or marker on an invader. When this antigen enters the body, the antibodies against it go into action, attacking and destroying it. A common example involves the immunity conferred by a vaccination: the body is deliberately exposed to a small, usually inactive or altered amount of a potentially harmful substance, such as the virus that causes polio. The body recognizes it as a harmful invader, even though it may have been altered enough to render it harmless. The immune system produces antibodies against the specific vaccine, and should a live, disease-causing virus of that type later invade the body, the antibodies will prevent it from doing any harm.

In people with allergies, the immune system fails to distinguish between harmful and benign foreign substances. Normally, our bodies simply process the harmless substances in food, air, medications and the like without our even being aware of what is happening. In people with allergies, however, the immune system goes into action against normally harmless substances, such as pollen, animal dander, and a wide variety of chemicals in food and the environment. The immune system makes different kinds of antibodies. The one that precipitates most allergic reactions is called IgE. Each allergic substance stimulates the manufacture of an IgE antibody that goes into action against only it; for example, the IgE for ragweed pollen does not "recognize" the antigen in animal dander or any other substance. People with allergies have many more IgE antibodies than normal, and these are unleashed whenever exposed to their specific antigens. Antibodies are attached either to *basophils,* a type of white blood cell, or *mast cells,* which line the airways, gastrointestinal tract, and skin.

When an IgE antibody finds the allergen it is programmed to counter, it signals the basophil or mast cell to release histamine and other chemicals into the surrounding tissue, resulting in the characteristic allergic reaction. For example, histamine released in the airways will cause tightening of the bronchial muscles and increased mucus secretion. If the histamine is released in the nasal passages, it can cause sneezing and a runny nose. In the skin, it can cause hives and itching. Abdominal cramps and diarrhea are common manifestations of histamine released in the gastrointestinal tract. The severity of the allergic reaction depends upon the level of specific IgE—the more IgE in the body that recognizes the antigen, the more intense the reaction.

Allergy-induced asthma is referred to as *extrinsic asthma.* It usually appears in early childhood, and may be accompanied by hay fever, eczema, food allergies, and other allergic conditions. There is often a family history of allergies and asthma; in fact, it is not unusual for several family members to suffer from extrinsic asthma. This type of asthma usually can be diagnosed by a careful history of asthma symptoms following exposure to the allergen. If this is inconclusive, the next step might be a challenge—that is, a patient will be deliberately exposed to a suspected triggering agent such as pollen or animal dander and then observed for signs of an attack. Skin tests also are useful in diagnosing the asthma and identifying triggering factors (see Chapter 6 for a more detailed discussion of this).

The less common form of the disease, *intrinsic asthma,* is not as closely associated with allergic disorders or a family history of asthma. Patients usually have normal IgE levels and negative skin tests. Intrinsic asthma generally appears in adulthood, and often is associated with other respiratory disorders, such as bronchitis or sinusitis. Frequently, the asthma will first appear following a viral upper respiratory infection. Since these patients usually do not have a family history of asthma, the diagnosis often comes as something of a shock. Peter Jenkins, a thirty-two-year-old lawyer who came to the National Jewish Center after four hospitalizations in less than two years, recalled his surprise when he first learned he had asthma.

"My asthma started with a bad cold that developed into bronchitis, which I just couldn't shake," he told us. "After a couple of weeks, I had increasing difficulty breathing. I would sit up almost all night, just trying to get enough air into my lungs. I had seen my doctor a couple of times, and he had prescribed antibiotics and medication to help me breathe, but I didn't get any better. I finally ended up in the emergency room after I started turning blue and was barely able to get a breath. Shortly after that, I found out I had asthma." Over the next few months, Peter experienced a number of attacks, several severe enough to send him to the emergency room.

"I knew that even the slightest cold could land me in the hospital," he said. "Finally, I decided to take a month off from work and come here to learn what I could do to avoid these severe episodes."

In intrinsic asthma, attacks also may be triggered by emotional stress, exercise, changes in the weather, and a host of other factors. This type of asthma is often more difficult to control than extrinsic asthma, and is not as likely to go into long periods of remission. Still, patients usually can identify the factors that lead to attacks, and take steps to either avoid or control them.

Sometimes patients will show characteristics of both the intrinsic and extrinsic forms, a condition referred to as mixed asthma. Typically, patients with mixed asthma may have hay fever or other allergic disorders, as well as a family history of asthma or allergies. The asthma may first appear during childhood, and as the patient grows older, the allergic triggering factors may subside somewhat. For example, a child who invariably had repeated asthma attacks during the fall hay fever season may find that the seasonal triggering factors ease off, but they may not disappear entirely. And other provoking factors may appear: although the earlier seasonal episodes may no longer predominate, factors like a cold, exercise, or emotional upset—triggers normally associated with intrinsic asthma—may actually cause more frequent attacks than were experienced in the past.

Who Gets Asthma?

Although certain factors such as heredity and allergies may increase the likelihood of asthma, it is impossible to predict whether a person will actually develop the disease. There are numerous examples of people whose parents and siblings have asthma, yet whose own airways are perfectly normal; there also are people who have no known risk factors who develop severe cases of the disease. Epidemiologic studies have turned up some interesting facts about asthma in various population groups. For example:

- Boys are more likely than girls to develop childhood asthma, but their symptoms are more likely to abate as they get older. Thus in adulthood, the disorder is about evenly divided between men and women.

- Asthma is more common in industrialized countries with cold climates than in agrarian societies with more temperate climates. There are exceptions, however; asthma is very uncommon among American Indians, whereas Trinidad has one of the world's highest rates of asthma.

• American blacks have a high prevalence of asthma, whereas the disease is rare in some areas of Africa.

Even though there are still many unknowns regarding asthma, better understanding of the disease and improved treatments now mean that most patients can learn to control it. This may not be easy; it requires careful attention to lifestyle, and the avoidance of triggering factors. Asthma patients require more medical care than average—they lose more days from work or school, spend more time in hospitals, and need to see their doctors more often than nonasthmatics. Like any chronic disease, asthma can be frustrating and lead to emotional problems and strained relationships. Despite the difficulties, most people with asthma can cope with the disease. Theodore Roosevelt is one famous asthmatic, but he is by no means the only one. We can find people with asthma in almost every profession and endeavor. Asthmatics include Olympic athletes, corporate executives, celebrities, scholars, as well as millions of average people pursuing jobs and rearing families. Dr. Reuben M. Cherniack likes to tell patients at National Jewish Center that "with proper understanding and medical treatment, almost all asthma patients can gain control over their lives. It's a hard disease," he adds, "but it's one you can live with." In the following chapters, you will learn specific steps taught to patients at National Jewish Center to help them take charge of their asthma—and their lives.

CHAPTER 3
Living with Asthma

It would be folly to minimize the impact that asthma can have on the lives of asthma patients and their loved ones. This becomes clear in chatting with patients at the National Jewish Center for Immunology and Respiratory Medicine. Although the asthma of these patients may be more severe than average, their experiences and feelings are typical. We have changed the patients' names, but all the following stories are real.

Susan Barclay

Susan is a lively, outgoing thirty-one-year-old mother of three from Ohio. When we met her, she had been at National Jewish for three weeks; and although she missed her family—there were pictures of her two daughters and baby son on almost every surface of her room—she was very enthusiastic about her progress.

"I first developed asthma when I was about six years old," she recalls. "I would end up in the hospital two or three times a year and I missed a lot of school, but my mother never babied me or let me think of myself as being different or an invalid. I was urged to play with other kids, run around, and keep as active as possible.

"When I was in high school, my asthma seemed to get worse at one point and I was put on steroids. I suddenly turned into a butterball, and that was hard. I hated being a fatty, and I really started to resent my asthma and feel sorry for myself. Then when I was about seventeen, the symptoms seemed to disappear. I got off steroids and started dieting to lose forty pounds. By the time I went off to college, I was trim and very pleased with myself."

Susan recalls her college years fondly. She went to school in Virginia, and was not only a top student but also a cheerleader and a member of the student government. Following her graduation, she worked for two years in her father's business and then "married the boy next door." Her first daughter was born a year later, and, as she puts it, "life was a bowl of cherries. I was absolutely on top of the world." Two years later, her second daughter was born. But about six months after that, on the heels of her twenty-seventh birthday, Susan's life took a drastic turn.

"I developed a bad case of flu, which I couldn't seem to shake," she recalls. "I was constantly coughing up lots of phlegm, and had trouble breathing, especially at night. So many years had gone by since I had had an asthma attack, at first it didn't even occur to me that the disease had come back. Then one night I woke up and thought I was suffocating—I simply couldn't breathe. My husband was terrified and called for an ambulance. It was then I realized that I was having a severe asthma attack."

Until that time, Susan had assumed she had simply outgrown her childhood asthma. She had worried that her children might be asthmatic, but both her daughters seemed perfectly normal. "I became very depressed when my doctor told me that you don't outgrow asthma, and that it frequently recurs during adulthood." Still, Susan was determined not to let the disease get her down. Her older daughter went to a cooperative nursery, and Susan taught there one day a week. She continued to run her household and care for two lively children. "But there would be days I could barely make it up and down the basement stairs lugging a basket of laundry. I was constantly catching colds from the children in my daughter's nursery school, and every cold meant a flare-up in the asthma. I would try to ignore the warning signs that an attack was coming on, and invariably I would end up in the emergency room. Finally, my doctor put me back on steroids. Almost overnight, my weight shot up. I remembered how miserable I had been as a fat teenager, and I wasn't going to let that happen to me again. I tried stopping the drugs, and wound up back in the hospital. Deep down, I knew that my asthma was getting worse—at times, it seemed that everything I touched or did would trigger an attack."

With her doctor's help, Susan attempted to keep a diary of attacks and possible triggering factors. "We had a professional company come in and clean the house from top to bottom. I got rid of all our feather pillows, rugs, and other dust-catchers. The one thing I could not part with was our German Shepherd—all of us loved that dog like a member of the family." Susan's doctor finally persuaded her to put the dog in a kennel for a couple of weeks to see if her attacks abated. "I was almost happy when they didn't," she related. The dog came home, and Susan's asthma continued to get worse. "I was back on steroids, and there would be days when I simply couldn't get out of bed. I hated to admit that the asthma was getting me down—I was so used to going from dawn to midnight without stopping."

The steroids made her ravenously hungry, and she continued to gain weight. "I couldn't fit into any of my clothes, and ended up having to shop in the fat lady department," she says. "I can't tell you how humiliating that can be. And my face was all puffy and moon-shaped."

After three years of battling her asthma, Susan again became pregnant. "The symptoms abated somewhat, and I was more diligent about taking my medication as prescribed, and also resting when I needed to." But after her son was born, her asthma attacks became more frequent and severe. That was when she decided to check into National Jewish.

"My family is very supportive, but I knew I couldn't go on as I was. I was sick most of the time, the drugs were making me impossible to live with and doing terrible things to my body. My doctor felt that if I could get away for a month or even longer and concentrate on getting the asthma under control, we all might be able to lead a more normal life."

When we talked to Susan, she was markedly overweight, and even though her face had the round moon-shape that is a characteristic side effect of long-term steroid therapy, her good cheer and enthusiasm shone through. At National Jewish, her medication was adjusted to minimize the side effects while providing maximum benefit in reducing the number of attacks. She was put on a moderate diet to try to lose some weight, and also started a daily exercise program of swimming and working out on exercise machines. At the time of our meeting, she had not had an asthma attack for ten days—the longest she had gone without an episode since the birth of her son. She was keeping a careful diary of symptoms, and extensive testing had demonstrated a number of triggering factors, including animal dander. "When I told my husband that, he made the decision for me—our dog Dan was going to go live with his brother's family. The kids would be able to visit him, we knew he would have a good home, and I would be free of one more triggering factor."

We again talked to Susan five months after she returned home. She had had a few asthma attacks, but nothing she could not handle. She was losing about a pound a week. "In another year, I might be able to get back into some of my old clothes," she joked. But in a more serious vein, she said: "The asthma has not gone away, and I know deep down it never will. But now I feel that I am in control of my life again. I don't try to be Superwoman anymore. My husband does more around the house, and the girls are learning to pick up after themselves. I don't like the fact that I have asthma, and at times I feel a bit sorry for myself. Still, I know that I could have diseases that are a lot worse."

Tom Johnson

Asthma was a new experience to Tom, a twenty-five-year-old graduate student from Pittsburgh. He had developed the disease about four months earlier, and even though it was relatively mild he decided to spend part of his vacation in Denver to make sure it did not get out of control. Although asthma was new in Tom's life, living with a chronic disease was not. About ten years earlier, he had developed juvenile—or Type I—diabetes.

"I was in the hospital for several weeks when I first got diabetes, and my parents finally took me to the Joslin Clinic in Boston," he related. Over the years, he had learned to manage his diabetes to the point where he seldom had problems related to it. "I learned what I had to do to lead a normal life," he explained. "If this meant taking three shots of insulin a day and measuring my own blood sugar two or three times a day, so be it. I felt I didn't have any choice—it was that or ending up dead at an early age."

He obviously was approaching his asthma with a similar attitude. While some might indulge in self-pity over being dealt such a cruel double blow, Tom had decided early on that "feeling sorry for myself or denying the facts wasn't going to help anyone, least of all me." In Denver, he was happy to learn that many of the life-style practices that made living with diabetes easier also applied to asthma. "I jog three or four miles a day," he said, "and the doctors here have encouraged me to keep this up. My diet doesn't need changing —I simply need to make sure that I don't eat anything that contains sulfites" (a color-preserving food additive that can provoke a life-threatening reaction in people with asthma).

As is so often the case, Tom's asthma came on the heels of a viral infection. Since infection also exacerbates diabetes, he knows he has to be particularly careful when he feels he is getting a cold, flu, or other such illness. "The safest thing for me to do is simply check into the hospital at the very beginning, before both the diabetes and asthma get out of hand." While this may seem drastic to people who do not have these diseases, Tom's doctors agree with his strategy. "If I can get the problem under control at the beginning, I may only be in the hospital for a few days. Waiting may stretch this to weeks."

During his stay in Denver, Tom also was undergoing tests to determine triggering factors. So far, he had found that cigarette smoke ("Luckily, I don't smoke, but now I will be more adamant about not letting others smoke around me"), animal dander ("My family has several cats, but I now have my own apartment—they can visit me instead of my visiting them"), and emotional stress seem to be triggering factors. The latter is the most worrisome to him. "It's hard to erase stress from your life when you are preparing for graduate exams or working on a thesis defense," he said. "I've been spending a lot of time with psychologists here, working out stress-management strategies." Books on his bedside table included *The Relaxation Response* and *Type A Personality*—a further indication of the determined manner in which Tom approached his health problems.

Tom might be called a model patient, but some doctors might worry about his almost too eager bravado. "There is no denying that asthma can make life difficult," one noted. "A cheerful, determined outlook is certainly a plus. But we also have to make sure that the determination does not carry over into self-denial."

In a follow-up conversation with Tom, he related that he felt his three-weeks' stay in Denver had been well worthwhile. "I learned what I needed to know about asthma in one concentrated time period. I now think I know what I have to do to keep both the diabetes and the asthma under control." He has had several relatively minor attacks, which he could control himself. He also has spent four days in the hospital when he caught a bad cold. "If I can hold such episodes to one or two a year, I will consider myself lucky," he says.

Richard Jacobs

When we met Richard, he was trying to convince a nurse that he should be allowed to skip his afternoon exercise session, pleading that he just wasn't feeling up to it. "I'd rather stay in my room and work on my stamp collection," he explained. She resisted his winning ways, and sent him off with a group of other youngsters to work out in the exercise room. In discussing Richard, she cited him as a typical example of a child whose asthma has become a focal point for considerable family unrest. "His parents mean well, but their opposing approaches to his health problems have not always worked to Richard's benefit," she explained. And Richard has not been above capitalizing on his family's concerns. "It's hard to resist his charms," she confessed, "and unfortunately, he pulls every trick in the book to get his own way."

Richard's charm is hard to escape—his impish grin, freckles, and mass of curly red hair make him look like the all-American kid next door. We were surprised to learn that he is 15 years old; his short stature and chubby build make him look much younger. He first developed asthma at the age of two, and he is one of those youngsters whose symptoms worsen during adolescence. Over the years he has missed a considerable amount of school time, but he has kept up with his grade.

Richard's asthma has had a profound effect on the entire Jacobs family. He readily admits that his parents "fight all the time" over his asthma and how it should be treated. His mother is very protective of her son, whereas his father thinks she babies him too much and that Richard is simply using his disease to get his own way. "My dad keeps telling me to grow up and stop acting like a baby," Richard relates.

Family counseling is an important part of Richard's treatment. His asthma is moderately severe, but doctors are confident that it can be brought under better control. For most of his life, Richard has been discouraged from engaging in exercise—only his father has tried to engage him in sports or other physical activities. "My Dad was a football player in college, and I think he would like me to play football, too." Richard explains. He related how his father had set up a dummy tackle in their back yard, and had been trying to teach his son to play football. What Mr. Jacobs did not realize was that years of steroid therapy, as well as his sedentary lifestyle, had weakened Richard's bones. "I busted my arm and that was the end of football," Richard explained, adding that the accident had resulted in a major dispute between his parents. "My Mom kept shouting at my Dad that she had told him I couldn't do anything like play football."

Instead, Mrs. Jacobs encouraged her son to concentrate on his stamp collecting and other hobbies that were interesting but not physically challenging. Richard has been put on an exercise program designed both to increase his stamina and to improve his self-image. At times, he resists exercising, but he also concedes that he was surprised to find out he could learn to swim. Although it is difficult for Mrs. Jacobs to agree to let her son participate in sports—not football, but swimming and other activities that will improve his physical fitness without endangering his bones—she now understands that physical inactivity is not in his best interest. By the same token, Mr. Jacobs has gained a better understanding of his son's disease, and has come to realize that it is a physical, not an emotional disorder.

Common Myths About Asthma

Most people with asthma do well, but many are hampered by persistent myths, some of which actually worsen the disease and make life much more difficult. Among the most common myths are the following:

Asthma is mostly psychological. This is one of the most persistent and damning of the myths surrounding asthma. The disease may cause emotional problems, and emotional stress may precipitate or worsen an attack, but psychological factors do not *cause* asthma. Sometimes parents think that a child deliberately provokes an attack of asthma to gain attention or to avoid a chore or other task. Sometimes an asthmatic may associate attacks with anxiety and take Valium or some other tranquilizer or sedative—medications that have no beneficial effect on the asthma itself, but which can be life-threatening because they actually decrease respiration and mental alertness at a time when just the opposite is needed.

Children outgrow asthma. Although symptoms may lessen or even disappear as a child grows older, the hyperreactivity of airways that is characteristic of asthma persists for life. This sensitivity can be demonstrated in pulmonary function tests. Frequently, people who had childhood asthma and seemingly outgrew it when reaching adulthood will suddenly resume having attacks after a bad cold or other respiratory infection. The triggering factors may change and the episodes may be milder (or in some instances, more severe) than in earlier years. Similarly, the episodes may be more or less frequent.

Asthmatics should avoid sports and other vigorous physical activity. Unfortunately, many asthmatic children are discouraged from participating in school sports and other activities. Overly protective parents may mistakenly fear that exertion will provoke an attack; coaches and teachers who do not know how to deal with asthma frequently refuse to let an asthmatic child participate, fearing they will be held liable if something goes wrong. In some instances, exercise may induce an asthma attack, but this usually can be avoided by commonsense preventive measures. (See chapter on Exercise and Asthma.) Regular exercise is an important part of the overall management of asthma because it improves lung function and helps the body make more efficient use of available oxygen.

Asthma can destroy the lungs. The lung changes that occur during an asthma attack are fully reversible, and cause no permanent lung damage. Although some asthmatics who persist in smoking cigarettes may go on to develop emphysema or other irreversible lung conditions, asthma does not cause these diseases. In very rare instances, chronic severe asthma can cause a form of persistent airway obstruction that is not totally reversible. In most cases, however, asthma is treatable and should not lead to respiratory impairment.

Asthma interferes with normal growth and development. Steroids, drugs which may be used to treat asthma, may interfere with growth; but asthma itself, unless exceptionally severe, does not. Many parents mistakenly fear that a diagnosis of asthma means that a child will develop a barrel-shaped chest and will not achieve his or her normal height potential. Steroids may stunt normal growth, but most children with asthma can be managed very well without needing steroids to the extent that they will interfere with growth.

CHAPTER 4

How to Tell If It's Really Asthma

An accurate diagnosis is an essential step in arriving at the best approach for treating asthma, and patients at the National Jewish Center can expect to undergo a battery of tests to establish that they do, indeed, have the disease. Sometimes people with breathing problems think they have asthma, only to learn that some other condition with similar symptoms is at the root of their difficulties. There are instances of people who are being treated for asthma, when, in fact, other conditions such as chronic bronchitis may be causing the difficult breathing. Even if there is no doubt that the patient has asthma, careful testing is essential to identify the factors that trigger an attack.

The symptoms that are hallmarks of asthma—shortness of breath, labored breathing, wheezing, increased mucus production, and coughing—also are characteristic of chronic bronchitis, cystic fibrosis, emphysema, and certain other lung disorders. In unusual cases, the problem turns out to be vocal cord dysfunction; this is a complex, usually psychological problem in which the person, often unconsciously, manipulates the vocal cords to mimic the sound of wheezing and hinder the passage of air into the bronchi. There are case histories at National Jewish of patients who had undergone years of asthma treatment who, in reality, did not have the disease at all, but instead had used their vocal cords to mimic asthma attacks.

Lung Function Tests

An accurate diagnosis of asthma requires that a doctor do a number of tests designed to give an accurate picture of how well the lungs are functioning. The first instrument that comes to mind when people think of breathing tests is the stethoscope. But in the case of asthma, this basic tool is not precise enough to give the physician a clear picture of what is happening in the respiratory tract. Lung function tests are needed to measure the severity of the disease. The most frequently performed lung function tests are usually done in the doctor's office using a spirometer, and at home with a peak flow meter.

Spirometry

This painless procedure measures the volume of air that can be expelled from the lungs, and the amount of resistance to airflow in the respiratory tract during expiration. In the opinion of Dr. Reuben Cherniack of the National Jewish Center, spirometry should be as routine as blood pressure readings for *all* patients.

The spirometer consists of a mouthpiece and tubing connected to a recording device with graph paper. The patient is asked to breathe in a variety of ways into the mouthpiece, depending on the specific function to be measured. The volume of air breathed in or out and the time required to do it are plotted on the graph paper. The tests may be done both before and after a dose of an inhaled bronchodilator to measure its effectiveness; before and after exposure to a suspected trigger; or before and after exercise. By comparing spirometry results at different visits against expected results for normal individuals, the physician can gauge the progress of the disease. Age, sex, and height also influence lung function—for example, a tall male under thirty can exhale more air at a faster rate than a short woman in her fifties—and must be taken into account when interpreting the results.

Lung Functions Affected by Asthma

Patients often have difficulty interpreting the results of lung function tests. The table on page 32 lists ten of the most common test values. The two most common functions measured by spirometry are the FVC (forced vital capacity) and FEV_1 (forced expiratory volume at one second). The FVC is the amount of air that can be forcefully exhaled after taking in a full breath. The FEV_1 is the amount of air that can be forcefully exhaled within one second, after taking in a full breath. (A related indicator is the FEF25-75, the mean or average rate of exhaled airflow during the middle of a forced expiration.) To measure FVC, FEV_1, and FEF25-75, the patient breathes normally through the mouth for several breaths. Then he or she takes a slow full inspiration and blows out the air as fast and hard as possible into the spirometer. The blowing should be done for at least six seconds. To obtain an accurate measurement, the test will be done three or more times.

The test results indicate the amount of work required for breathing—that is, how much effort the lungs and respiratory muscles, particularly the diaphragm, must make to overcome resistance from both natural and disease factors. For example, friction within the trachea and the bronchi create an inherent resistance to airflow; in asthma, bronchospasm and mucus buildup add to this resistance. For this reason, the FEV_1 is lower than normal in asthma patients.

Table 1

Terms Used to
Describe Pulmonary Function

Tidal Volume (TV) The amount of air flowing in and out of the lungs during a normal breath.

Inspiratory Capacity (IC) The maximum amount of air that can be inhaled after a normal expiration.

Total Lung Capacity (TLC) The amount of air in the lungs after a maximum inspiration.

Vital Capacity (VC) The maximum amount of air that can be exhaled after a maximum inspiration.

Functional Residual Capacity (FRC) The amount of air left in the lungs at the end of a normal expiration.

Expiratory Reserve Volume (ERV) The additional amount of air that can be exhaled after a normal expiration.

Residual Volume (RV) The amount of air left in the lungs after a maximum expiration. The residual volume may be higher than normal in asthma patients.

Forced Vital Capacity (FVC) The greatest amount of air that can be rapidly and forcefully exhaled after a maximum inspiration.

Forced Expiratory Volume in One Second (FEV$_1$) The amount of air exhaled in one second during a forced expiration following a maximum inspiration. This measures air flow resistance and is often below normal in asthmatics.

Maximum Mid-expiratory Flow Rate (MMF, also FEF25-75) The average rate of air flow during the middle half of a rapid, forced expiration.

Home Testing

An alternative way of measuring the expiratory flow at home is by a peak expiratory flow meter. The device consists of a tube and indicator, either a dial or vertical scale. (See Table 2, *How to Use a Peak-Flow Meter.*) The patient blows as hard and fast as possible into the tube and reads the velocity of air expelled in liters per minute. A drop of more than 15 to 20 percent below the usual (base line) reading is a sign of increased airflow resistance. The flow meter helps the patient recognize increased airflow resistance in the early stages, spot any specific triggers of an attack, and assess whether a particular medication is effective in relieving obstruction. The physicians at the National Jewish Center note that taking a series of readings with a peak-flow meter is especially valuable in detecting obstruction and assessing the effectiveness of a treatment program.

Table 2
How to Use a Peak-Flow Meter

Before using your peak-flow meter, read the instruction manual that comes with the device. Use the meter at a consistent time relative to your treatment each day. The standing position is the best one to use for the test. Establish a baseline reading by blowing several times into the meter when your breathing is unimpaired. The best of these readings becomes your baseline.

1. Return marker to zero.
2. Hold the device so that your fingers do not obstruct movement of the marker.
3. Inhale a maximum breath, set mouthpiece between teeth, and seal it with lips.
4. Exhale immediately with a maximal "huff."
5. Read and record your best effort. Depending on your physician's guideline, a drop of 20 percent below baseline may indicate the need for medication. A drop of 50 percent that does not improve with medication is a signal to call your physician.
6. To clean the device, immerse the mouthpiece in a vinegar solu-

tion or disinfectant three times a week. Alternatively, wipe mouthpiece with alcohol to clean. Periodically soak the entire device in a mild detergent for thirty minutes.

Challenge Testing

People with mild asthma may have symptoms only when exposed to a particular trigger such as animal dander or certain food additives. Although some offending substances may be spotted during peak expiratory flow testing at home, challenge testing with spirometry is a more accurate means of determining whether the lungs are hyperreactive to particular substances or activities. In a bronchial challenge test, the patient is deliberately exposed to a suspected asthma trigger, and the effects on lung function are measured. Spirometry is done before and after the challenge, and a drop of 20 percent in the FEV_1 indicates that the lungs are hyperreactive to the substance or activity. National Jewish doctors stress the importance of blinded challenges to ensure that the patient's reactions are unbiased. The patient will be tested with both a placebo and the actual substance, and will not be told which is which.

Most often, challenge tests are done to confirm a diagnosis of asthma in cases in which there is some doubt, and to identify specific triggering factors. Challenge tests also are done to assess the degree of airway hyperreactivity and the effectiveness of specific medications to prevent or reverse the bronchospasm. Before doing a bronchial challenge, the patient is instructed to abstain from medications and other substances that may alter the results (see Table 3). Challenge tests should be carried out in a medical setting with personnel capable of handling an emergency should one arise. Challenge tests are not recommended for patients with severe bronchoconstriction because of the risks involved and the fact that the results are not likely to be as meaningful as in patients who can breathe normally. Following are some of the more common challenge tests.

Table 3
Patient Preparation for Bronchial Challenge Tests

Following are the recommended times, from the last dose of medication or other factors, before undergoing a bronchial challenge test.

SUBSTANCE	HOURS OF ABSTINENCE
Inhaled bronchodilators	
Short-acting beta-agonists (e.g., isoprotenol)	4
Longer acting beta-agonists (e.g., albuterol)	12
Atropine and anticholinergics	12
Oral bronchodilators	
Liquid theophylline	12
Short-acting theophylline	18
Aminophylline	18
Intermediate-acting theophylline	24
Beta-agonists (e.g., terbutaline)	8–24
Long-acting theophylline	48
Antihistamines	48
Hydroxyzine	96
Cromolyn sodium	6–48
Steroids	Maintain constant level
OTHER FACTORS	
Smoking	2–6
Caffeine (e.g., coffee, tea, cola)	6
Exercise	2

SUBSTANCE	HOURS OF ABSTINENCE
Viral infections	2–4 weeks
Vaccinations	3–6 weeks

From Pathophysiology and Physiologic Assessment of the Asthmatic Patient, by Charles Irvin, PhD., and Reuben Cherniack, M.D., in *Seminars in Respiratory Medicine: Asthma, Part One.* Robert J. Mason, M.D., Editor. Thieme Medical Publishers, New York, 1987.

Methacholine Challenge

A *methacholine* (or, less commonly, a histamine) challenge is done to confirm a diagnosis of asthma. Bronchial smooth muscles have receptors for acetylcholine, a neurotransmitter of the autonomic nervous system. Methacholine is structurally similar to acetycholine, and the bronchial muscles respond to both substances in a similar manner. Usually asthma can be diagnosed simply by noting improvement in airflow following inhalation of a drug that dilates the constricted bronchial muscles. A methacholine challenge can determine the degree of lung reactivity. All lungs eventually respond to methacholine, but in an asthmatic, the response will occur at a lower-than-normal dosage.

Before the challenge, a baseline FEV_1 will be determined. Typically, the patient will then inhale a placebo, and the FEV_1 will be measured. Then the patient will inhale increasingly larger doses of methacholine, and lung function will be measured after each administration. The point at which reactivity is noted indicates the degree of lung reactivity.

Exercise Challenge

Most people with asthma will eventually develop exercise-induced bronchospasm, but the degree of exercise tolerance varies greatly among them. At one time, it was expected that the more severe the asthma, the less physical activity could be undertaken. Studies at National Jewish have discounted this—some patients with very mild asthma will start to wheeze with only minor exercise, while others with more severe disease will have a much higher tolerance. During an exercise challenge, the patient will walk briskly on a treadmill, or pedal an exercise ergometer, at speeds fast enough to push the heart rate to 85 percent of its safe maximum potential rate. Typically, the patient will exercise for ten minutes. Lung function is measured during the exercise and, since many patients experience a delayed reaction to exercise, again ten to fifteen minutes after stopping.

Aspirin

About 8 to 14 percent of asthmatics experience an idiosyncratic response to aspirin. National Jewish doctors advise adult patients to avoid aspirin and nonsteroidal anti-inflammatory drugs, especially if they seem to provoke asthma flare-ups. But for asthmatic patients who may need aspirin therapy —it is the most commonly used drug to treat arthritis, for example—an aspirin challenge may be useful in determining whether they can safely use the drug. The challenge typically starts with a low dosage and works up to 650 mg, or two regular tablets.

Metabisulfite

Metabisulfite, more commonly referred to simply as *sulfite,* is a food preservative commonly used to prevent browning of potatoes, cabbage, or apples, and to preserve the colors of fresh vegetables. It is also found in dried fruits, as well as beer and wine. Some asthmatics experience a hypersensitive reaction to sulfites, but not all people with the disease react to it. Sulfite challenges may be carried out to demonstrate whether a person can safely eat foods containing sulfites. Doctors at National Jewish have found that about 15 percent have positive reactions in a placebo-controlled test, but that when the same patients are given double-blind challenges— neither the patient nor the testers aware of what substance is being administered—only about half of these demonstrate true reactions.

In the past, challenges to tartrazine, or Yellow Food Dye #5, have been done at National Jewish and other institutions, but more recent studies have failed to demonstrate their usefulness for most patients. Tartrazine testing is now done on a very limited basis, if at all.

Occupational Irritants

Bronchial challenges to demonstrate reactivity to possible asthma triggers in the workplace are difficult to do in a clinic or lab setting because it is impossible to duplicate the exact environment. Ideally, the challenges should be carried out at the workplace; if this is impossible, the tests should be done with the actual substances that a person works with. For example, if chemicals in a paint or varnish used in the patient's workplace are suspected as provoking the asthma, the doctor should make sure that the tests are carried out in a blinded fashion using the actual products.

Specific Antigens

Inhaled bronchial challenges using specific antigens are sometimes done, but more often with children than with adults. Usefulness of these tests is limited by a wide variety of abnormal responses to inhaled antigens. Some patients will have an immediate response; others may not have a response for several hours, and still others may react immediately and again later on. Late responses can be severe and prolonged, lasting for several days. Thus, National Jewish doctors caution that bronchial challenges with specific antigens should be approached with care and under careful supervision.

Beyond the Basic Measurements

Measurements obtained through basic spirometry are not always conclusive indications of asthma being the one and only cause of respiratory problems. For example, the low FEV_1 and FVC found in asthma may also be seen in other obstructive diseases such as emphysema, and in conditions that result in a stiffening of lung tissues such as pulmonary fibrosis. To get a more complete evaluation, the physician may order tests that measure lung volumes. To measure absolute lung volumes, the patient must breathe gas containing a trace of neon or helium which is diluted by the gas in the lungs for measurement, or breathe while sitting in a special device known as a body plethysmograph. The total lung capacity is the amount exhaled plus the amount of air remaining in the lungs. These categories can be further broken down (air in the lungs at the end of a normal expiration, air inspired and expired in normal breathing, and other measurements) to get a more precise idea of lung function.

In both asthma and emphysema, the total lung capacity is larger than normal; however, in asthma this is because air is temporarily trapped within the lungs because of bronchospasm, whereas in emphysema it is caused by a permanent loss of lung elasticity. Basic spirometry measuring only the FEV_1 and FVC might not pick up any improvement even after a dose of inhaled bronchodilator has reversed the spasm and the patient feels better. More sensitive determination of lung volume could pick up a reduction in trapped air after a forced expiration, confirming the subjective improvement.

One of the ways to measure lung volume is by body

plethysmography. In this test, the patient sits inside an air-tight chamber breathing through a mouthpiece leading to the outside air supply. At a specific moment at the end of a normal expiration, the tester closes a shutter within the breathing apparatus, trapping air that is left in the patient's lungs. The patient is then instructed to hold his hands against his cheeks and pant, breathing gently but rapidly against the obstruction. The resulting compression and decompression of the lungs, and changes in pressure within the chamber, are used to calculate lung volume.

Lung volume is also measured by spirometry using either helium, which is not normally present in the lungs, or pure oxygen which "washes out" a certain amount of nitrogen with each breath. By calculating the dilution of gases, the physician can measure various compartments of lung volume and arrive at a total.

Measurement of Blood Gases

Blood gas testing measures the pressure of dissolved oxygen and carbon dioxide in the blood. These pressures are directly related to the actual amounts of gas and are an important indication of lung function. Normally the blood takes in oxygen and discards waste carbon dioxide in the alveoli. During an asthma attack, obstruction interferes with the normal exchange and the oxygen level falls, depriving cells of a vital nutrient. In a very severe attack, the carbon dioxide level may rise, and if it becomes too high, the blood becomes acidic.

Physicians at National Jewish Center stress the need for measuring—in addition to blood gas levels in the arterial blood—the pressure of oxygen in the alveoli compared to that in the surrounding pulmonary capillaries; this is called the $P(A-a)O_2$. Normally, these values are quite similar; air enters the alveoli, and oxygen goes right into the bloodstream. During an asthma attack, oxygen distribution in the lungs becomes very uneven and causes an abnormal spread in these numbers. This value, together with a drop in arterial oxygen, is a very sensitive indicator of peripheral airway obstruction. (Peripheral airways make up a very small percentage of resistance to airflow and may not lead to a decrease in the FEV_1.) Treatment at this stage can prevent a more serious attack.

Blood gas measurements may be taken when the patient has no symptoms, or during an attack or an exercise test. Complex relationships between increased oxygen demand during exercise, blood levels of oxygen and carbon dioxide, and blood acidity can indicate trouble spots in the cardiovascular system as well as the respiratory tract. To obtain an arterial blood sample, the physician or lab technician first checks for good circulation to the radial artery in the wrist by applying pressure to each side and asking the patient to clench and open the fist. If color returns soon after pressure on the artery is removed, there is adequate circulation for the test. A needle is then inserted into the radial artery or, less frequently, an artery at the inside of the elbow or in the groin. Because the artery may be harder to find than a vein, the tester may have to insert the needle more than once. Arteries also run deeper than veins and the procedure is more painful than having a blood sample taken from a vein.

Sometimes gases in expired air are collected simultaneously with arterial blood. If this is called for, the patient simply breathes into a specially prepared spirometer or rebreathes air into a small bag.

Distribution and Diffusion of Gases

Closely related to blood gas measurement is testing to see how evenly oxygen is distributed in the lungs and how fast it moves into the pulmonary capillaries. Obstructed airways in an asthma attack result in irregular filling and emptying of the alveoli, rather than the normal in-unison movement of air in and out.

To measure gas distribution, the patient breathes in pure oxygen, and the expired nitrogen concentrations are measured to calculate the level of oxygen concentration. In the Single Breath Nitrogen Test, the patient takes two maximum inspirations and then exhales fully. Then, he or she takes a maximum inspiration of 100 percent oxygen and breathes out very slowly as far as possible. In the Nitrogen Washout (Multiple Breath Technique) Test, the patient breathes pure oxygen for seven minutes, exhaling into a bag or spirometer. At the end of this time, he or she takes a maximum breath out.

Gas diffusion testing measures how fast a small amount of carbon monoxide crosses from the alveoli into the surrounding capillaries. An abnormally slow rate of diffusion usually indicates a loss of alveolar surface area. The diffusion capacity is usually normal in asthma but low in emphysema. Carbon monoxide is preferred over oxygen for this test because of its greater affinity for combining with hemoglobin, which makes interpretation of the results easier. In the D_LCO (diffusing capacity of carbon monoxide), the patient takes a deep expiration, then a single deep inspiration from a bag or spirometer containing air mixed with carbon monoxide and helium. He or she then holds that breath for ten seconds and breathes out fully into a collecting bag. The amount of carbon monoxide and helium in the collecting bag are measured. The concentration of helium in the expired gas measures the air within the chest that dilutes the inhaled helium. The carbon monoxide in expired air is reduced both by dilution and transfer to hemoglobin.

Pressure-Volume Testing

Pressure-volume tests measure lung elasticity and help determine whether lung disease is *obstructive*, as in asthma and emphysema, or *restrictive*, as in pulmonary fibrosis; and measure the degree of reversibility. In asthma, loss of elasticity is temporary and reversible; in emphysema, the loss is permanent.

The pressure volume-test is as follows:

- No food or drink is permitted for three to four hours before the test.

- The examiner inserts a small deflated balloon through the nose. It is equipped with pressure sensors and attached to plastic tubing.

- The patient swallows the balloon into the stomach and air is injected to confirm the position.

- The balloon is then pulled back up into the esophagus where pressure will be measured, and then the balloon is inflated.

- The patient is instructed to breathe in different ways into a spirometer. Changes in pressure during the breathing maneuvers are plotted against changes in volume. A decrease in lung elasticity is noted if it takes a smaller than expected change in esophageal pressure to bring about a specific change in volume.

Sleep Studies

There are two different asthma problems that may develop during sleep. Up to 75 percent of asthmatic patients experience reduced pulmonary function during sleep. In some people, the asthma worsens during sleep despite their taking medications as instructed and getting along fine during the day. The second abnormality is a cessation of breathing, a condition called *sleep apnea* and one that is not limited to asthmatics. Sleep apnea is relatively rare, but of increasing interest to physicians because of recent research indicating it may be linked to sudden death while sleeping.

Nocturnal asthma studies are designed to determine how much a person's asthma worsens during sleep, and also to study the effectiveness of different medications and strategies in preventing nighttime worsening. The testing requires that the patient be observed while sleeping on at least two nights, and in some instances, up to seven nights. The initial studies can be carried out in an ordinary hospital setting; more formal studies requiring extensive monitoring and equipment will be done in a sleep laboratory.

In routine nocturnal asthma studies, spirometry is done before and after bedtime treatments and upon awakening in the morning. In addition, if the patient awakens during the night, spirometry measurements are taken.

Other determinations of lung function depend upon the situation, and may include measurements of oxygen saturation while using an earpiece; arterial blood gas measurements; and electrocardiographic monitoring of the heart's rate and rhythm. The patient also will be observed for various symptoms such as wheezing, coughing, gastric reflux, or general restlessness. If the patient is taking theophylline medication, blood levels of the drug will be measured before he or she goes to sleep, at any awakenings during the night, and upon waking up in the morning.

If these baseline sleep tests indicate nocturnal asthma, additional testing will be carried out on succeeding nights to determine the causes and most appropriate treatments. Sometimes the problem can be solved by increasing the nighttime medication or shifting a daytime dosage to bedtime. For example, a patient who takes a daily steroid medication may take it in the evening instead of the morning. If the problem is related to gastric reflux (see Chapter 8), the patient will be given appropriate medications and the head of the bed will be elevated on four- to six-inch blocks. The patient will then be observed during the night to see if these measures prevent the asthma's worsening. Sometimes the best solution is simply for the patient to set the alarm to wake himself up so he can take an inhaled medication during the night.

If these conservative tests and techniques fail to reveal the cause of and provide relief for the nocturnal asthma, more elaborate polysomnographic tests in a sleep laboratory may be required. This involves sleeping while attached to various monitoring devices, which include:

1. Sleep staging leads. These are small sensors that are applied around the head, eyes, and chin to determine the quality of sleep and the length of time spent in different sleep stages.

2. Heart monitors. Electrocardiogram leads are attached to the chest to record the heart's rhythm during the night.

3. Ear oximeter. This is a small clothespin-like device that is attached to the ear to continuously measure the oxygen level in the blood. The amount of light transmitted through the earlobe to the probe is converted mathematically into the blood's level of oxygen saturation.

4. Respiration monitors. Coiled springs are stretched around the chest and abdomen to measure expansion and contraction during breathing.

5. Air-flow sensors. Small sensors are placed in the nose and mouth to measure the amount of airflow through these passages. These sensors also detect a cessation of airflow, which may happen during sleep apnea.

6. Esophageal sensor. In some instances, a small balloonlike device will be placed in the patient's esophagus to measure the breathing effort.

Most patients with nocturnal asthma do not require elaborate sleep-laboratory studies. Those that do often insist that they will not be able to sleep while hooked up to all the monitors, and question whether the results will have any meaning. However, the sensors used are small, and after a few minutes most people are hardly aware of them. Every effort is made to make the patient as comfortable as possible, and most manage to fall asleep without difficulty.

CHAPTER 5

Early Warning Signs of Asthma

Although many people contend that an attack of asthma comes on without warning, in fact there are almost always signs of an impending episode. If these early warning signs are recognized in time, and proper preventive action is taken, a full-blown episode often can be forestalled completely or at least minimized. The problem is that the warning signs may be so subtle that many people do not recognize them.

Part of the asthma education program at National Jewish focuses on helping patients become more attuned to their bodies and to signs of an impending asthma attack. (See Table 4 on Early Warning Signs of Asthma.) Many patients are so accustomed to wheezing and to the tightening of their airways that even these symptoms will be ignored until the attack has progressed to a severe or even life-threatening stage. Patients are encouraged to keep a diary of each episode, logging in any possible exposure to triggering factors and any signs that may have preceded an attack. (See Wheezing Episode Form—Table 5.) They can then use this diary for more effective self-care of their asthma. For example, if an asthmatic patient realizes that in the hours or even day or two before an attack he or she invariably feels moody and tired, or experiences a slight chest tightness, these signs can serve as an indication to increase medication or take other preventive action.

Table 4
Early Warning Signs of Asthma

Knowing what your early signs of asthma are is an important part of asthma self-care. Pediatricians at National Jewish developed the following checklist of warning signs to help children become more attuned to their particular disease. Adults as well as children may experience these symptoms.

SYMPTOM	YES	NO	SOMETIMES
Breathing slows down			
Feel funny in chest			
Get headache			
Feel spacey			
Eyes look glassy			
Get upset easily			
Feel sad			
Get excited			
Feel nervous			
Have watery eyes			
Feel clammy			
Feel feverish			
Get scratchy throat			
Have dry mouth			

SYMPTOM	YES	NO	SOMETIMES
Have itchy throat	_____	_____	_____
Cough	_____	_____	_____
Sneeze	_____	_____	_____
Have runny nose	_____	_____	_____
Get pale	_____	_____	_____
Heart beats faster	_____	_____	_____
Am tired	_____	_____	_____
Want to be alone	_____	_____	_____
Get quiet	_____	_____	_____
Feel weak	_____	_____	_____
Slow down	_____	_____	_____
Get mopey	_____	_____	_____
Feel droopy	_____	_____	_____
Have dark circles under eyes	_____	_____	_____
Feel grumpy	_____	_____	_____
Head plugged up	_____	_____	_____
Feel restless	_____	_____	_____

On the spaces below, add any early signs for you that are not listed above:

_____

_____

_____

Table 5
Wheezing Episode Form

Name _____

It was hard for me to breathe today _____
(Date)

While I was _____
(What were you doing?)

At _____
(Where were you?)

My peak flow was _____

These are the signs of asthma that I observed:

_____
_____
_____
_____

This is what I did:

(Check what you did)

Kept doing what I was doing _____

Just hoped it would go away _____

Got away from precipitant _____

Got upset _____

Rested _____

Drank something cold _____

Drank something warm _____

Took shower _____

Used humidifier _____

Used nebulizer (make one check for each whiff): _____

Took pill _____

Asked an adult for help _____

Saw doctor _____

_____

_____

_____

Later, my breathing got OK in _____ minutes or _____ hours.

　　　　　　　　　　　(How many?)　　　　(How many?)

My peak flow was _____.

_____

Not all patients experience the same warning signs, and the signs may vary in a given individual. A warning sign may appear only a few minutes before an attack, and at other times there may be several hours or even a few days during which a person will experience hints of an impending flare-up. To help young patients recognize warning signs for what they are, National Jewish pediatricians compiled a check-list of common warning signs, which are presented in Table 4. Although originally developed for children, the checklist is useful for patients of all ages to enable them to review warning signs that may have appeared before an attack, and take appropriate preventive action in the future.

What to Do When Warning Signs Appear

Successful asthma self-care pivots around knowing what to do to prevent an asthma attack from progressing to a crisis stage. The earlier the preventive action is taken, the better the chances of success. This is why early warning signs are so important. Specific steps that should be taken include:

Increase fluid intake. Fluids are needed to prevent dehydration, provide added moisture for the lungs, and keep the mucus thin. Giving a child a glass of fluid to drink will also help focus attention on something other than wheezing and other symptoms, and thereby ease anxiety and promote relaxation. All people with asthma should drink six to eight glasses of fluids a day, and more during a flare-up.

Relax. By stopping what you are doing and taking a few minutes to rest and relax, you can ease the stress and emotional tension that may be contributing to the symptoms.

Practice breathing exercises. Diaphragmatic or deep breathing (described in Chapter 17) helps prevent air from becoming trapped in the lungs. It also allows better control of breathing and prevents overbreathing or hyperventilation, which can exacerbate asthma. Postural drainage exercises may be needed to help clear mucus and prevent it from plugging the airways.

Check on lung function. During an asthma attack, patients breathe more rapidly. By counting how many breaths per minute you are (or a child is) taking, you can get a better indication of what is going on. Under normal circumstances, adults breathe about ten to fifteen times a minute; a child takes twenty to twenty-five breaths, and babies take thirty to forty. Prolonged rapid breathing in a baby or young child with asthma is an indication to seek medical help. At National Jewish, patients also are taught how to monitor their own respiration function using a peak flow meter. Changes in lung function can be detected with a peak flow meter even before symptoms become obvious. By monitoring these changes, a person can learn when extra medication is needed, and can seek medical help early before a crisis develops.

Take medication as instructed by your doctor at the first sign of an attack. All too often, people delay taking medication early in an attack, thereby increasing the chances that the problem will get out of hand. Many times, people will be reluctant to use an inhaler in public, or will try to hold in coughing for fear of drawing attention to themselves. Children especially may be reluctant to interrupt play or other activities to take medication. The importance of early preventive treatment cannot be overemphasized. Although a person may be self-conscious about using an inhaler in a public place, the chances are that others will not even notice. More importantly, appropriate extra use of the inhaler may prevent the need for an emergency room visit or even a hospitalization.

CHAPTER 6

The Child with Asthma

Asthma is the most common chronic childhood illness, afflicting between three and five percent of all children in the United States. For many, the disease is mild and causes only occasional problems. For others, it can be so severe that it disrupts normal life for both the child and the family, and at times is even life-threatening. Most cases of childhood asthma fall between these two extremes. The child will experience more than average sickness and may require occasional hospitalization or trips to the emergency room during acute or prolonged attacks. But between episodes, the youngster can carry on with normal activities, provided he or she follows an appropriate medical regimen.

In reality, however, many asthmatic children, including those with mild forms of the disease, grow up convinced that they cannot run and play or even go to school like other youngsters—that they are in some way handicapped. When these youngsters come to the National Jewish Center for Immunology and Respiratory Medicine, they often are surprised to learn that once they know how to control their asthma, they can function just like other children. Regardless of the severity of the disease, virtually all children with asthma and their families can benefit from learning as much as possible about the disease and its control.

In about half of all cases of childhood asthma, the disease makes its first appearance before the age of three. In young children, the disease is more common in boys than in girls. After puberty, however, the numbers even out, and among teenagers and adults the incidence is somewhat more common among females than males. Asthma that begins in infancy or during adolescence is more likely to be severe, with frequent attacks, than asthma that arises during childhood.

Many parents mistakenly assume that a diagnosis of childhood asthma inevitably means that the youngster will develop irreparable lung damage, such as emphysema, or that he or she will be more susceptible to heart disease. This is not true; the tightening of the breathing passages that occurs during an asthma attack is temporary, and in most instances does not cause lasting damage if treated properly. The emotional scars on both the child and other family members are likely to be more permanent than any physical disabilities.

An asthma attack can be a very frightening experience at any age, but especially when it occurs in a child. The wheezing, congestion, coughing, and difficult breathing characteristic of asthma is often more pronounced in a child than in an adult; and because a child's airway passages are smaller, an episode may progress more rapidly to a medical emergency. Thus, both the youngster and the parents should be attuned to early warning signs and take immediate steps to prevent an attack from progressing to a crisis stage.

Helping the entire family cope with asthma is a major treatment goal at the National Jewish Center, where a large proportion of the patients are children. Youngsters who come here often are expected to stay for several weeks, and, during that time, to develop more effective methods of controlling their asthma—methods aimed at helping them resume a normal life-style. Visitors to the center often remark that it does not seem like a hospital, and in many respects this is true. The center's complex includes classrooms, exercise rooms, and playgrounds; parts of the children's wards more closely resemble boarding-school dormitories than a hospital. The children appear active and attentive; few give the impression of being sickly. At times, it is hard to believe that most of these children have long histories of severe asthma—the average age of onset is about two—and that most have been in and out of hospitals several times a year.

Of course, most children with asthma do not require treatment at a special hospital like National Jewish, but all can benefit from the unique approach practiced at this center. Simply becoming more observant and learning how to relate symptoms with triggering factors are vital steps in controlling a child's asthma. As noted by Dr. Robert C. Strunk, Acting Director of Pediatric Medicine, "Just the fact that we can observe the child twenty-four hours a day for a given period (usually four weeks) means that we can spot factors that may otherwise go unnoticed."

Even though a child with asthma receives more medical care than the average healthy youngster, many obvious factors still may escape observation. The child's regular doctor is likely to spend only a few minutes with the patient during a routine office visit. During a typical hospital stay, the child is apt to be quite sick, and this is no time to observe daily routine. Thus, most of the information-gathering is left to the parent, usually the mother. "Obviously, most mothers are well aware of what is happening to their children, but they usually do not know how to interpret what they are observing," Dr. Strunk explains. "At a place like this, we have well-trained nurses and other professionals who are aware of the many nuances of asthma, so we can learn a tremendous amount about the child and his or her disease in a relatively short time."

General Approach

Children referred to National Jewish usually stay about four weeks; those with severe, complicated asthma may be there for several months. To provide the maximum benefit in the time available, the Center has developed a systematic approach aimed at determining the best treatment. Thus, all children can expect to undergo:

- Detailed pulmonary function testing
- Allergy, exercise, and provocative testing to identify precipitating factors
- Adjustment of medication based on twenty-four-hour observation of wheezing patterns related to specific triggering factors and response to medications
- Rehabilitation, including exercise conditioning, recreational therapy, sports and life-style counselling, and evaluation and recommendations regarding school performance.

Since the ultimate goals are both to control the asthma and to encourage the child to lead as normal a life as possible, the program at National Jewish goes far beyond diagnosis and treatment. For example, children are expected to attend classes even while undergoing treatment. "Most of these children are capable of doing very well in school," Dr. Strunk notes, "and most are at grade level, even though the average patient has missed up to 25 percent or more of school. But we see many youngsters whose asthma is totally out of control, and they simply are unable to function normally in school. Some have dropped out completely; others are performing far short of their capabilities. We spend a good deal of time communicating with teachers and school personnel, advising them on how best to manage the child in school and how to deal with asthma attacks."

A Stay at National Jewish

All children who come to National Jewish come via a doctor's referral. Some come because of unusual features of their lung disease and/or side effects of medications, and hope that evaluations at the Center will be able to provide additional insight. Others are referred simply because they are not responding to treatment as would be expected. Perhaps it is because the child is not receiving medication as instructed, or because he or she is being exposed to undetected or ignored precipitating factors at home. Since asthma can put tremendous strain on all members of the family, there often are emotional and behavioral problems that make following an effective treatment program difficult or impossible to implement on an outpatient basis.

Typically, when a child checks in at the Center, the first three days or so are spent in intensive orientation and information-gathering. The patient will undergo a number of medical tests to confirm the diagnosis of asthma and to determine its severity, as well as to evaluate the effectiveness of current treatment. If possible, the parents are expected to be on hand during these initial three days so that they can be interviewed by doctors, nurses, social workers, and others who will be working with the child. During this orientation and information-gathering phase, hospital staff members will try to learn as much as possible about all facets of the child's disease: What triggers an attack? In what ways has the child's asthma affected family relationships? How is the child doing in school? Does the youngster play with other children? Does exercise trigger an attack, and if so, what kinds of activities are most likely to be tolerated?

Intensive education directed at helping the patient learn

how to control the asthma is a major component of the National Jewish program. Asthma education for both the child and parents begins during the orientation program. "We have found," Dr. Strunk explains, "that noncompliance is closely related to the level of understanding." For example, teenagers often rebel at taking needed medications or needlessly expose themselves to triggering factors. But by becoming involved in an intensive educational program with peers and sympathetic nurses and counsellors, they can better understand the mechanics involved and realize that they can control their asthma by following certain precautions and medical regimens. Under these conditions, compliance improves markedly.

Establishing the Diagnosis

By the time a child is referred to National Jewish, the diagnosis of asthma is usually well-established. However, this is not always the case for children with breathing difficulties, and it is important to rule out other lung disorders. Whenever asthma is suspected, specific tests should be performed to make sure that the problem does not have other causes. For example, chronic bronchitis—characterized by inflammation of the bronchial tubes, wheezing, coughing, and excessive mucus secretion—is frequently mistaken for asthma. Although chronic bronchitis is more common in adults, especially heavy smokers, than it is in children, it still should be ruled out before a doctor assumes that the problem is indeed asthma. Other specific problems that should be ruled out include:

Inhaled foreign objects. As any parent knows, children are always putting things in their mouths, and occasionally an object may be inhaled into the windpipe or lungs. This usually causes a fit of coughing and choking during which the object is expelled. Sometimes, however, the object will become lodged in the windpipe or a bronchial tube. If it is small enough and positioned in such a way that some air still can pass into the lungs, it will not cause asphyxiation, but can produce wheezing, coughing, labored breathing and other symptoms of asthma. Therefore, before making a diagnosis of asthma, chest X rays during deep inspiration and expiration should be taken to determine whether an obstruction is producing the symptoms. The suspected asthma may turn out to be a swallowed object; everything from safety pins to bottle caps and parts of toys have been turned up by these diagnostic X rays. Occasionally, bronchoscopy—a test in which a tube with special lights and viewing devices is inserted into the airways—will be needed to study the airway anatomy and to rule out obstruction from a foreign body or abnormal branching of the airway. A local anesthetic is used to minimize discomfort.

Birth defects. A number of congenital defects, including heart defects, can cause difficult breathing. Often there are other symptoms that will point to the real problem, but sometimes the symptoms will closely mimic those of asthma. X rays and other diagnostic tests are needed to make a positive diagnosis.

Bronchiolitis. This disorder, which is caused by a viral infection, involves inflammation of the bronchioles and is most common in babies and young children. It causes wheezing, coughing, and difficult breathing; it also may be accompanied by a fever. Generally, bronchiolitis occurs once, whereas asthma has recurrent episodes. In children with a personal or family history of asthma and allergies, bronchiolitis may be a forerunner to asthma.

Cystic fibrosis. This is an inherited disease affecting the glands that secrete sweat and mucus. The sweat is excessively salty and the mucus is very thick and profuse. Typically, the lungs become clogged with thick mucus, leading to increased susceptibility to bacterial infections; there is also fast, labored breathing, and wheezing and coughing—symptoms which may be mistaken for those of asthma. A sweat test to measure the amount of salt in the sweat will point to the correct diagnosis.

Pneumonia. This is a general term for lung inflammation that leads to a buildup of fluid in the air spaces, resulting in difficult breathing. Pneumonia may be caused by an infection, which may be bacterial, viral, or fungal; or, less commonly, by chemical damage to the lungs such as inhalation of poisonous gases. Coughing and difficult breathing, often accompanied by fever, are common symptoms of pneumonia. Since pneumonia can be life-threatening in a baby or person weakened by other illness, early diagnosis and treatment are important. A chest X ray will detect the abnormal fluid buildup.

Croup. Croup is usually distinguished by its barking cough, but sometimes it is mistaken for asthma. Croup usually occurs following a cold. Typically the child will wake up with a harsh cough and labored, noisy breathing. If the child is having marked difficulty in breathing, or his or her lips have a bluish tinge, immediate medical care should be sought. However, most cases of croup can be handled at home. Taking the child into a warm, steamy room, such as a bathroom with a hot shower running, usually will relieve the cough and make breathing easier. As with asthma, an attack of croup can be frightening for both the parents and the child. Crying and anxiety can increase the difficulty in breathing; calm, quiet assurance from the parents, coupled with guidance from a doctor on lessening the symptoms, help ease the anxiety.

Epiglottitis. The epiglottis is the lid-like structure that closes off the trachea, or windpipe, to prevent swallowed substances from invading the airways. In young children, the epiglottis sometimes becomes inflamed and swollen, usually as a result of a respiratory infection. The problem may come on suddenly, and is often accompanied by a high fever. Drooling accompanied by difficult breathing, lethargy, and anxiety are common symptoms. Since closure of the windpipe can lead to death, emergency medical treatment is vital. The child should be taken to an emergency room, and, if necessary, an artificial opening in the trachea (a tracheotomy) may be needed to restore breathing.

Swollen tonsils and adenoids. The tonsils and adenoids are masses of lymphoid tissue located, respectively, in the back of the throat and in the nasopharynx area. Their function is to help protect the body from infection; sometimes they become inflamed and enlarged, and can lead to wheezing and difficult breathing. In the past, many children routinely had their tonsils and adenoids removed, especially if they had frequent sore throats and colds. This is no longer done as a routine matter; tonsillectomies are now performed only if the glands are clearly diseased. Swollen tonsils and adenoids may cause some difficulty in breathing but they do not cause asthma, nor will their removal cure it as some people mistakenly assume.

Psychological and Social Problems

Although asthma is a physical rather than psychological disease, it often leads to emotional problems that make treatment more difficult. Thus, dealing with psychological and social issues is an integral component of the program at National Jewish. During the orientation period, patients undergo psychological as well as physical testing, and in some instances it turns out that the emotional problems become the major focus of treatment.

"We find that some of the children are severely depressed," Dr. Strunk explains. "They have simply given up. These youngsters are more likely to die of their asthma than are children who are determined to fight on. For these children, recognizing and treating their depression is vital."

Other youngsters come with serious behavioral problems. Some use their asthma to gain attention. Acting out in regard to illness-related issues is particularly common. These children often know what they should do to control their asthma, but sabotage their own treatment to gain attention, often unconsciously. Noncompliance is frequently encountered. "Sometimes, a child will go so far as to hide medicine under his or her tongue," Dr. Strunk says. "Others will take too much medicine or they will feign symptoms. Some have even subconsciously learned how to control their vocal cords to make a noise that sounds like asthmatic wheezing. Although this vocal cord dysfunction is more common in adults than children, it does occur. Sometimes it is subconscious, but in many of these children, it is a conscious act."

Some youngsters may use their asthma to avoid going to school and assuming other responsibilities. For others, it may become an attention-getting device. In many instances, a child's psychological problems are closely intertwined with those of the parents. Not uncommonly, a child will quickly learn that if he or she has an asthma attack, it will stop or prevent parents from quarreling between themselves. Instead of focusing on the underlying problems in their marriage, the parents will shift their attention to the child's health problem. In a way, the child is using the asthma to keep the parents from fighting, and perhaps even to hold a shaky marriage together. In other instances, a child may deny the severity of the asthma to avoid negative reactions to illness from peers, parents, or teachers.

A child's asthma will often become a focus for parental strife. Typically, the mother—who usually bears the burden of caring for the asthmatic child—will become overly protective, while the father will contend that the child is being coddled too much, and that what is needed is a firm hand. Grandparents may become involved in "taking sides." "We have encountered children who are masters at manipulating their family members, friends, teachers, and others to do their will," a National Jewish social worker explained. "All too often, everyone has been afraid to say 'no' to the child. This can lead to discipline and behavior problems in a healthy child, and in this respect, an asthmatic youngster is no different."

National Jewish has a special unit devoted to treating psychological or social problems. "Understandably, many parents resist having their children switched to this unit," Dr. Strunk comments. Quite often, they feel that their children's problems reflect their own shortcomings. For others, it is easier to come to terms with the fact that their child has severe asthma rather than confronting deep-seated emotional problems that originate with the parents and their relationship to each other. "It is important to understand that the psychological problems are as real as the physical aspects of asthma," Dr. Strunk says, and that treating one without the other is not likely to do much good. Here, the adolescent, or May Unit, which is devoted to psychological as well as medical treatment, is an integral part of the entire program. "We stress that it's all part of the same treatment program, and only the emphasis is different," Dr. Strunk explains.

Rehabilitation

Rehabilitation and discharge planning begin during the initial orientation period. Regardless of the severity or duration of the asthma, the overriding objective for all National Jewish patients is the same; namely, to return them to their home communities with the asthma under control, and with the ability to lead as normal a life as possible. This includes going to school, exercising, and engaging in other normal activities.

Many of the children who come to National Jewish have had their activities severely restricted because of their asthma. In many instances, the restrictions have been imposed more as a result of misunderstanding and of complex emotional factors than because of the severity of the disease. For example, asthma attacks frequently occur in association with exercise. If running and playing with other children causes an attack of asthma, chances are that the youngster will avoid the activity. A vicious cycle sets in: As a child becomes increasingly sedentary, tolerance of exercise is likely to decrease further. Parents and teachers are reluctant to encourage the child to exercise for fear of precipitating an attack.

"Many of the children we see score very low in physical fitness," Dr. Strunk says, "not because of their asthma, but because they are extraordinarily sedentary." Very often, the child is unaware of just how restrictive the asthma has become. The youngster will concentrate on nonphysical pastimes such as music, reading, stamp collecting, computer games, and the like. "When we ask these youngsters if asthma is imposing restrictions on their lives, they often will say 'no,' " Dr. Strunk says. "But closer questioning will reveal that they and their friends spend most of their time playing computer games or watching TV rather than participating in physical activities." Thus, getting children into a manageable exercise program is an important part of the National Jewish rehabilitation program. "Many children who never thought they could run or participate in sports are surprised when we show them that they can be more active," Dr. Strunk says. (This is discussed in more detail in Chapter 10.)

Performance in school is another area that is likely to suffer among asthmatic children. Typically, children with asthma miss a good deal of school—those referred to National Jewish have been absent from school 25 percent or more of the time. When they are in school, these children may be discouraged from participating in normal activities, particularly gym and physical education programs. Teachers may feel that they are not qualified to deal with a child's asthma, or may be reluctant to assume this responsibility. Not uncommonly, a child's behavorial and emotional problems will be particularly pronounced in a school setting. School-age patients at National Jewish are expected to attend school, and the center's social workers and other staff members spend a good deal of time observing them in classroom settings. As Dr. Strunk notes, "We see youngsters who do a lot of acting out in school, making their asthma appear a good deal worse than it really is." Part of a child's discharge and rehabilitation planning includes detailed reports and telephone conferences to help teachers in his or her home community. Follow-up studies comparing school absenteeism have found that attendance usually improves by 50 percent after a child undergoes the treatment/rehabilitation program.

Dr. Strunk and other National Jewish staff members attribute a good deal of this improvement to group dynamics. "When we talk to patients and their parents after a stay here," Dr. Strunk explains, "the one thing they remember most is meeting other children with asthma. Simply knowing that they are not alone, that others have the same problem and may be a lot worse off, comes as a real revelation. For the first time, many of these youngsters are encouraged to go outside and play baseball or other games, to go to school and participate in other normal activities. Suddenly, they realize that having asthma is not such a bad thing. They will say, 'Yes, I've got it and I don't like it, but things could be a lot worse.' Once we have been able to instill this lesson, the major part of the battle is won. We can fine-tune their medication and show them more effective ways of managing their asthma, but the most important accomplishment has been in overcoming the psychological barriers."

Environmental Factors

The emphasis on dealing with psychological factors related to asthma should not be misconstrued to imply that they in some way cause the disease. As repeatedly stressed in this book, asthma is a physical disease that may be exacerbated by emotional factors, but its origins are not psychological. An important part of asthma control lies in identifying and, as much as possible, eliminating any environmental factors that provoke asthma attacks. Some of these may be obvious; if a child begins wheezing whenever exposed to a cat or to cigarette smoke, for example, it is clear that these are triggering factors and should be avoided. "It is surprising how many parents of asthmatic children continue to smoke," notes Dr. Robert Mason, Chairman of Medicine at National Jewish.

Unfortunately, many triggering factors are not so obvious, and some that are may be impossible to avoid. In some instances, allergy shots to desensitize the patient may be in order. In most cases of severe asthma, a combination of avoiding triggering factors and taking medication is necessary. Even so, the more a patient can avoid the triggering factors, the less the amount of medication needed for control.

At National Jewish, considerable time and testing are devoted to the identification of triggering factors. This may entail skin tests to identify allergens, as well as challenges during which the youngster is deliberately exposed to small amounts of a suspected triggering factor and then observed for responses to it and to medication.

Not uncommonly, removing a triggering factor from an asthmatic person's environment meets with considerable resistance. Pets are at the top of the list of items people are reluctant to part with. Dr. Strunk recalls one family that had tried to introduce a cat into a household with an asthmatic child. Over the next six months, the child was hospitalized more than twenty times because of severe asthma attacks. The youngster's physician could not understand why the child's asthma had taken such a turn for the worse. The family had neglected to mention the presence of a cat; after the doctor found out about the animal and persuaded the family to give it to a neighbor, the child's asthma improved dramatically. (For a detailed discussion on identifying and eliminating triggering factors, see Chapter 7.)

"People often ask me if there is anything that a child with asthma cannot do," Dr. Strunk remarks. "The list is relatively short: He or she cannot have a dog, cat, bird, or other furry or feathered pet. The child may not be able to run a marathon or participate in other endurance sports, but activities that require short bursts of energy, such as baseball, basketball, tennis, swimming, or sprints, are fine."

CHAPTER 7

Removing Factors
That Provoke Asthma

Some people with asthma will tell you that virtually everything—exercise, the weather, strong perfumes, tobacco smoke, dust, pollen, even laughter and dozens of other things —can trigger wheezing and even an attack. While this may be an exaggeration, it is true that there are a large number of factors that can provoke an asthma attack. These vary from person to person, and sometimes differ from time to time within an individual. One of the most important steps in taking control of asthma involves identifying triggering factors, and then making a concerted effort to either avoid them or to reduce their ability to provoke an asthmatic reaction.

At National Jewish, patients undergo careful questioning as well as tests to identify factors that provoke their asthma. (See the Sample Questionnaire in Table 6.) After identifying precipitating factors, every effort should be made to eliminate them from the asthmatic's environment. The answer varies from case to case, and is often complex. For some supersensitive people, there may be no way in which every triggering factor can be removed from the environment. In such instances, allergy shots or immunotherapy to desensitize the person to the precipitating factor may be considered. (See section on allergy shots later in this chapter.) Learning how to use anti-asthma medication also can help minimize the effects of many triggering factors. Following are major categories of the factors that provoke asthma, and suggestions for minimizing their effects.

Table 6

Sample Questionnaire to Identify Asthma Triggers

Many things can trigger an asthma attack; a number of known factors are listed below. Check the ones that are most likely to cause your asthma. List any additional triggers in the spaces provided, then go back and circle the five most likely to cause an attack.

---

1. **Airway Irritants**

_____ Aerosol Sprays

_____ Odors

_____ Smoke

_____ Dust

_____ Air Pollution

_____ Paint

_____ Perfume

2. **Animals**

_____ Dogs

_____ Cats

_____ Birds

_____ List any others:

_____

_____

_____

3. **Changes in Breathing**

_____ Sneezing

_____ Coughing

_____ Laughing

_____ Crying

_____ Choking and Gasping

_____ Hyperventilating

_____ List any others:

_____

_____

_____

4. **Exercise**

_____ Running

_____ Jumping

_____ General Exercise

5. Foods and Drugs
   - _____ Nuts
   - _____ Shellfish
   - _____ Aspirin
   - _____ List any others:
   - _____
   - _____
   - _____
   - _____

6. Health and Physical Condition
   - _____ Fatigue (Overtired)
   - _____ Colds or Infections
   - _____ List any others:
   - _____
   - _____
   - _____

7. Just Get It
   - _____ Night
   - _____ Day

8. Molds

9. Plants
   - _____ Trees
   - _____ Grass and/or Weeds

_____ Pollen
_____ List any others:
_____
_____
_____

10. Weather and Elements
    - _____ Wind
    - _____ Weather Changes
    - _____ Rain and/or Snow
    - _____ Hot/Cold Temperatures
    - _____ High Humidity
    - _____ Low Humidity
    - _____ List any others:
    - _____
    - _____
    - _____
    - _____

11. Emotions
    - _____ List any feelings that may trigger an attack:
    - _____
    - _____
    - _____
    - _____

Allergies

Many people with asthma are afflicted with related conditions, most commonly hay fever and other allergies. Some unfortunate people have a long list of substances that provoke an allergic reaction; others may be allergic to only one or two items, and still others may not realize that their symptoms are caused by allergies. Often they go from doctor to doctor with a long list of hard-to-pinpoint symptoms, such as headaches, chronic tiredness, irritability, stomach upsets, joint pains, itchiness, and others. Physicians are increasingly attuned to testing for allergies when confronted with symptoms that have no obvious physical cause. But there still are many instances in which allergies go undetected.

There is little doubt that allergies can play havoc with day-to-day life. People who do not have allergies often are insensitive to those who do. They find it hard to believe that a commonplace substance or object that does not bother most people can make an allergic person acutely uncomfortable, or even very ill. Often they think the allergy sufferers are putting on an act, or are simply using allergic reactions as an avoidance or attention-getting tactic. Of course, nothing could be further from the truth. The misery produced by allergic reactions, which range from vague feelings of unrest to the more familiar itching, runny nose and eyes, and difficult breathing, is as real as that caused by any other physical ailment.

Some of the common misunderstandings regarding allergies can be traced to the fact that they are poorly understood even by doctors, and are frequently difficult to document. In general, an allergy is any hypersensitive reaction to a specific substance, or allergen. Such reactions occur when the body's immune system, which is designed to protect us from harmful foreign invaders such as viruses and bacteria, goes into action by producing antibodies against harmless substances, or allergens. (Table 7 lists some of the more common allergens.) The reaction may be in the form of allergic rhinitis, characterized by sneezing; tearing and burning eyes; nasal stuffiness or discharge; and/or itchiness around the nose, eyes, and mouth. Allergies also may affect the skin. Eczema, or allergic dermatitis, is a common example. In rare, extreme cases, a person who is acutely hypersensitive to a substance will experience a generalized reaction that, if not reversed, can lead to anaphylactic shock and even death. A generalized allergic reaction is always a medical emergency; the most common examples are acute hypersensitivity to bee stings, penicillin, and certain other drugs, and to specific foods. Asthmatics may be particularly vulnerable to anaphylaxis; for example, there have been reports of death among asthma patients who unwittingly ate foods that had been treated with sulfites.

Table 7
Common Allergens

Inhalants

  Pollens

    Early spring: Trees

    Late spring–early summer: Grasses

    Late summer and fall: Weeds (i.e., ragweed)

  Molds/Fungi spores: mushrooms, grain molds, mildew and many others

  House dust/dust mites

  Animal dander

  Feathers

  Kapok

  Cottonseed, flaxseed

  Pyrethrum and other insecticides

  Industrial chemicals

Ingested Substances

  Specific foods (see lists in Chapter 11: *Food and Asthma*)

  Penicillin and other specific drugs

Injected Substances

Bee and other insect venom
Specific drugs

Allergens are among the most common culprits in triggering asthma, although there are some asthmatics who do not have allergies and, of course, only a fraction of the 35 million Americans with allergies develop asthma. The allergens may be inhaled—dust, molds, pollen, and animal dander are common examples—or ingested in food or drink.

As noted earlier, the histamine and other substances produced during an allergic reaction cause inflammation and swelling of the air passages, as well as increased mucus production. In addition to histamine, the immune system produces a number of other substances that can affect the airways. For example, leukotriene (LTE_4) causes smooth muscles to contract, thereby contributing to the bronchial spasm characteristic of an asthma attack. Leukotriene is slow to take effect, and when it does go into action, its effects may persist for hours or even longer. Thus, some people may not relate consumption of a certain food with their asthma, because the attack may not occur until many hours later. It is much easier to make the connection when a person experiences almost immediate wheezing after coming in contact with, for example, a cat or another allergen. *Prostaglandins,* body chemicals that can produce inflammation and numerous other effects, and a number of other naturally occurring substances, also may play a role in allergy-induced asthma.

In addition to allergens, there are a number of substances that produce idiosyncratic responses in some people. Common examples include aspirin, food additives, and inhaled irritants (especially tobacco smoke). Perfumes and other odors, pollutants, and industrial chemicals are other common examples of irritants that provoke asthma in sensitive individuals. These irritants differ from allergens in that they trigger asthma without provoking an immune-system response. Studies have found that people with asthma will have a stronger reaction to a smaller amount of an irritant than will a nonasthmatic. It is not known why asthma causes this idiosyncratic response, but it is believed that a number of factors are involved to make asthmatics more vulnerable to these nonspecific irritants. For example, the irritant may produce inflammation, which increases lung twitchiness and can trigger an asthma attack. It also should be noted that an asthmatic is more likely to be sensitive to nonspecific irritants than other individuals.

Identifying Allergens

There are a number of different tests that can be administered to track down specific allergens. Since allergy testing can be costly and time-consuming, and the results less than perfect, patients are often advised to keep a careful diary and observe their reactions to various suspected allergens before undergoing tests. Very often, a person knows only too well the substances that provoke a reaction. In other instances, careful questioning by an allergist or other health professional experienced in this field can point to suspected allergens. A careful clinical history is much more important than a battery of tests. Significant questions include:

Do your symptoms worsen at specific times of the year? Hay fever—the popular term for allergies to ragweed and other plants that produce airborne pollen—is the most familiar of the seasonal allergies. People who are allergic to molds usually notice that their symptoms are worse during damp, humid weather, or at night, because that is when mold spores are most prevalent. Many people with hay fever find that their symptoms disappear after the first frost in the fall. The time at which the symptoms occur often points to the culprits. For example, someone who has a flare-up of symptoms in the early spring may be allergic to tree pollens. Others who cannot tolerate mowing the lawn or picnicking on the grass may be allergic to grass pollens.

Do certain places make your symptoms worse? A person who is plagued by symptoms while at school or work, but not at home, should investigate chemicals, molds, or other substances that may be present at the school or workplace. However, their reactions may be delayed and thus difficult to associate with triggering factors. Some substances in the workplace may cause a reaction at night, for example. Asthma that improves on weekends or during vacations suggests that the provoking factors may be at work. If symptoms appear after a trip to the zoo, a farm, or a household in which there are furry or feathered pets, suspect an allergy to animal dander.

Do you wake up with symptoms? People who are allergic to animal dander or to certain fibers—such as kapok, which is used to stuff furniture, pillows, toys, and mattresses—may wake up wheezing or with other symptoms. Sometimes nocturnal asthma can be traced to allergens in the bedroom. For example, a thorough investigation may reveal animal dander, molds, or other allergens in a bedroom air conditioner, or an accumulation of dust or dust mites in a mattress, or other unsuspected culprits.

Are your symptoms worse while indoors, and relieved by going outside? If so, household dust or dust mites may be the problem. No matter how meticulously a house is cleaned, a certain amount of dust is inevitable. House dust is produced by the inevitable breakdown of common household materials; you can see the particles suspended in a sunbeam. The dust also may harbor microscopic mites, which provoke asthma symptoms in some people. People who are allergic to house dust and dust mites often have symptoms year-round, but especially in the winter when the furnace is constantly blowing out dust-laden air. They may experience a worsening when cleaning house or emptying a vacuum cleaner. Cats and dogs also stir up house dust—another reason why these pets should be barred from an asthmatic's home.

Can you associate symptoms with certain foods or restaurants? Food allergies are often suspected but may be difficult to track down, especially because so many foods contain a number of hidden ingredients. An elimination diet followed by specific food challenges may be helpful in identifying (or ruling out) suspected food allergens. (For a more detailed discussion, see chapter 11.)

Do certain odors, such as those in a particular soap, cosmetic, or other such substance, provoke symptoms? Irritant reactions to ingredients in perfumes, hair preparations, soaps, skin lotions and other cosmetics are very common, but often overlooked. Some asthmatics often will notice a worsening of symptoms when they linger near a department store cosmetics counter, or when are in a beauty salon or barber shop. Room deodorants, scented toilet paper and other such products also may cause wheezing or other symptoms. These substances are considered irritants rather than known allergens.

Do the symptoms often occur on the heels of a headache or other minor aches and pains? People with asthma often are sensitive to aspirin, but many do not associate the painkiller with flare-ups of the disease. Aspirin is found in many medications, so asthmatics should carefully check the ingredient lists. Also, people with aspirin sensitivity should avoid nonsteroidal anti-inflammatory drugs, such as ibuprofen and other medications in this class, which are used for arthritis, menstrual cramps, headaches, and other pain or inflammatory disorders.

Testing for Allergies

Although relating symptoms to exposure often is sufficient to identify allergens, a number of tests may be used to confirm the relationship. These tests include:

Prick or "scratch" skin tests. These tests, which are similar to the familiar skin tests for TB, may be used to diagnose allergies to inhaled substances or foods. However, the skin tests to inhaled antigens are much more reliable than skin tests to foods. An extract of the suspected allergen is prepared and sterilized, and a small amount is then applied to the skin in one of two methods: (1) A drop of the extract is placed on the skin, usually on the arm or back, and the skin is pricked with a needle; or (2) a small scratch is made on the skin and a drop of the extract is placed over it. About twenty minutes later, the skin will be examined for any reaction. If the person being tested has antibodies against the substance, there will be a wheal, or hive. Since only a very small amount of extract enters the skin using the scratch or pricking techniques, a person will have to have a relatively large number of circulating antibodies to show a reaction. When the extract is injected further into the skin (intradermal testing), a reaction can be produced with a smaller number of antibodies than with the scratch tests. Intradermal tests are much more nonspecific and clinically less useful than prick tests. Individuals may have a positive reaction to an intradermal test which, if not associated with symptoms or natural exposure, is probably not clinically important.

A positive reaction to skin testing indicates that a person has antibodies against the substance, but it does not necessarily mean that the allergen will produce asthma symptoms. In testing for inhaled allergens, the more pronounced the skin reaction, the more likely a person is to have asthma symptoms. This is not necessarily true for foods—a person with only a small skin reaction may have severe asthma symptoms, while others who develop large hives from the test may eat the food with no other noticeable symptoms. Results also can be misleading if large amounts of extract are used; the resulting skin reaction may be from irritation rather than from actual antibody-mediated sensitivity.

To ensure that signs of sensitivity are not suppressed or masked by medication, patients undergoing skin tests are advised not to take certain medications for varying periods beforehand. Specifically, National Jewish patients are instructed not to take oral Atarax or Vistaril for four days before the test, or oral Actifed, Benadryl, Chlor-Trimeton, Dimetapp, Drixoral, Trinalin, Tagamet, or Zantac for three days.

Oral tolerance challenges. These tests are performed to determine sensitivity to a number of ingested items, especially aspirin and sulfites, and, less commonly, tartrazine (Yellow Food Dye #5). The patient is instructed to take specific amounts of these substances, and then to measure lung function with a spirometer at designated times. The tests are designed to learn whether there is an association between asthma symptoms and these common, closely related substances. To determine aspirin sensitivity, for example, the patient will take increasing amounts of the painkiller, beginning with 75 mg and then 325 mg and finally 650 mg. Since the refractory period following aspirin ingestion may last up to seventy-two hours, there is a three-day interval between each challenge. People who have experienced asthma attacks within twenty-four hours of taking aspirin should not undergo a challenge unless it is done under close medical supervision in a special asthma care clinic or unit. If there is lingering doubt as to whether aspirin is causing asthmatic reactions, a placebo challenge may be indicated. This entails giving a patient aspirin for some of the challenges, and a placebo or "sugar pill" at other times. The patient will not be told which he or she is receiving, to provide an unbiased test result. Since about 20 percent of asthmatics are sensitive to aspirin, National Jewish physicians urge all patients with the disease to avoid aspirin and related anti-inflammatory drugs. An oral challenge may be useful, however, to confirm whether a person with arthritis or another condition normally treated with aspirin can tolerate the drug.

Metabisulfite sensitivity is also common among asthmatics, who are advised to avoid foods containing this preservative. In some cases, an oral tolerance challenge may be carried out to determine whether this is an unnecessary restriction.

Tartrazine, or Yellow Food Dye #5, is another common substance that is chemically related to aspirin, but not as likely to produce asthma symptoms. The challenge to this food dye is similar to that of aspirin: The patient will be given increasing amounts of the substance in successive days, followed by spirometry. If lung function drops by 20 percent or more, it can be assumed that the substance being tested is causing an asthmatic response, even though there may be no obvious wheezing.

Elimination diets. In tracking down a food allergy, an elimination diet is often prescribed. This entails consuming a limited diet of foods that usually do not produce allergic reactions; and then adding suspect foods one by one and observing whether they provoke symptoms. This is similar to the oral challenges for drugs. Only one food at a time is tested, and several challenges of the same food may be attempted. This can be a slow, arduous process, especially if a person has numerous food sensitivities. (For a more detailed discussion, see Chapter 11.)

Blood tests. Several blood tests may be used to help determine whether a person has allergies, but these are neither as accurate nor as specific as the skin tests. A complete blood count will indicate whether a person has an abnormally high number of a type of white blood cells called *eosinophils*. A 3 percent or higher elevation in eosinophils may indicate that a person has allergies. Another blood test can measure the level of IgE; a high result may indicate the presence of allergies.

RAST test. RAST, which stands for radioallergosorbent test, is a biochemical study using radiation to detect IgE antibodies against specific allergens. A blood sample is taken and sent to a laboratory where the blood is exposed to allergens and then studied under a special radiation device. A high level of antibodies indicates a good possibility of sensitivity against a particular substance, but a normal or low reading does not necessarily rule out an allergy. This test tends to be expensive, especially if a number of different allergens are being tested, and it is no more accurate than properly done skin tests.

Cytotoxic blood tests. These tests have become increasingly popular in recent years thanks to promotion by food faddists and others who are not necessarily trained in diagnosing and treating allergic disorders. A blood sample is taken and, while the white blood cells are still alive, they are exposed to allergen extracts. The idea is that if the white cells are damaged or destroyed, it is an indication that the person is allergic to the substance being tested. However, the test has no medical or scientific value. A reaction of white cells in a test tube does not necessarily reflect what happens in the body. Food components undergo many changes before entering the blood; exposing white cells to a food extract may be quite different from exposing the cells to a substance that has been digested. Researchers have found that substances that destroy white cells may not produce any allergic symptoms, while others that appear to have no effect on these cells can cause marked responses. National Jewish physicians stress that all patients, including asthmatics, should avoid cytotoxic tests. Certainly, they should not alter therapy on the basis of these tests, which are not accepted as scientifically valid by the medical community and researchers.

Added Warning

A word of warning about allergy testing in general. Unfortunately, many people with suspected allergies fall victim to unscrupulous practitioners, many of whom are not physicians or qualified to diagnose or treat allergies. This can be particularly dangerous for asthma sufferers. Skin and challenge tests must be performed with care to ensure against exposing a person to a large dose of an allergen, which may result in a serious asthma episode. The tests are often expensive, and unless performed and interpreted by properly trained laboratory personnel or physicians, the results can be false or misleading. Inaccurate testing often results in a person going on a needlessly restricted diet. Questionable positive results also may be used to persuade a person to undergo unnecessary and expensive desensitization treatments. In any event, a person with suspected allergies should check with his or her physician before undergoing any tests or treatments, and even then should make sure that the laboratory and physician are well-qualified to diagnose and treat allergic disorders. If in doubt, a patient can check with the American Academy of Allergy and Immunology, 611 East Wells Street, Milwaukee, Wis., 53202, for the names of qualified allergists.

Allergy Shots

Sometimes the treatment of allergy-induced asthma is simply a matter of avoiding whatever precipitates the reaction. This can be relatively easy if only a few avoidable allergens are involved. A person who is allergic to nuts or chocolate, two examples of common food allergies, usually can manage to avoid foods containing these ingredients without great difficulty. Similarly, a person who is bothered by cats or other dander-shedding furry animals usually can forego living with them, and either avoid households that have such animals or take preventive medication before visiting them.

Unfortunately, avoiding more pervasive allergens such as pollen, molds, or household dust may be more difficult and excessively restricting of normal activities. Antihistamines and other medications to control symptoms may be prescribed; this strategy is particularly useful in dealing with hay fever or other seasonal allergies. (See Chapter 16.) Some people try to solve the problem by moving to another part of the country. The Arizona desert has long been touted as a haven for allergy sufferers, and some people who move to a different climate do achieve relief. However, this is often short-lived. Even the desert has a large number of pollen-producing plants and trees, and allergy sufferers often learn that they have simply traded one set of triggers for another. In addition, people who have moved to Arizona and other such places tend to bring their favorite plants from home. Lawns, trees, and flower gardens filled with plants that are not native to the area now blossom in places like Phoenix and Tucson.

When it is difficult or impossible to avoid or control triggering factors, immunotherapy, or desensitization, may be the best solution. This treatment is lengthy and can be expensive; thus it usually is not recommended for people with mild, seasonal symptoms, such as flare-ups that occur only for a short period and can be controlled with minimal medication, or for people who can easily eliminate the offending substance from their environment.

Immunotherapy, often referred to as allergy shots, entails giving injections of small amounts of the allergen over a period of time to gradually desensitize the body to it, thereby preventing an allergic response. Not all allergies can be treated in this manner; the shots seem to work best against molds, pollen, insect venom, or house dust. Food allergies do not respond as well, and are not usually treated by desensitization.

Anyone embarking on immunotherapy should expect to continue the shots for two to five years, and in some instances even longer. As a rule, the shots, which are purified extracts made up of the allergens, are given once or twice a week, but occasionally may be given several times a week at first to achieve more rapid results. Once the maintenance level is reached, however, injections are given at three- to four-week intervals.

In the beginning, only a very minute amount of the allergen is given. The extract dosage is gradually increased by very tiny amounts, usually .05–.10 milliliters a week. The idea is to help the body build a tolerance to ever-increasing amounts of the allergen until eventually the person can be exposed to the amount normally found in the environment without experiencing symptoms. When this point is reached, the shots may be continued for a few more months, and then gradually tapered off until—if no symptoms recur—they are eventually stopped altogether.

Allergy shots do not work for all patients. After a year or so, most allergists will evaluate a patient's progress; if no benefits are seen, the shots should be stopped and other approaches tried to control the symptoms. Since asthma has many triggering factors in addition to allergens, immunotherapy alone usually will not control the disease. But it still may be helpful for asthmatics who invariably suffer symptoms when exposed to unavoidable allergens.

Care must be taken in administering the shots, because even a small overdose can provoke a severe reaction. This is why most allergists recommend that the shots be given in a doctor's office, and that the patient stay long enough, at least twenty minutes, to determine whether there will be a serious response. If the shots are administered elsewhere, whoever is giving them should know what to do if an emergency arises.

Adverse reactions to the shots usually occur within twenty minutes, but in some unusual situations the reaction may be delayed for twelve or even twenty-four hours; thus it is vital that the patient and family members know how to recognize and deal with signs of a reaction. Although rare, there have been instances in which patients have died of ana-phylactic shock after receiving an allergy shot. In one recent case, a young man left his allergist's office before the twenty-minute waiting time was up because he did not want to be late for work. He apparently suffered a reaction in the park-ing lot, but instead of seeking immediate help, he got into his car, where he was later found dead. It should be stressed that on the whole, allergy shots are safe if they are administered by trained medical personnel who can determine the proper dosage and also take proper action if an emergency arises. Most reactions are local, generally a hive around the injection site. But people with asthma are more likely than non-asthmatics to develop systemic reactions, such as wheezing, difficulty in swallowing, widespread hives and itching, gastro-intestinal symptoms, fainting, or, in extreme cases, circulatory collapse and death. Adrenalin or antihistamines can reverse a systemic reaction if administered promptly.

Allergy-Proofing Your Home

Although it may be impossible to eliminate all environ-mental allergens and airway irritants from your home, there are a number of relatively simple steps that can be taken to minimize their number and concentration. Keeping a home as free as possible from unnecessary dust, molds, and other allergens often entails considerable effort; mothers of asth-matic children often complain that they spend a dispropor-tionate amount of their time vacuuming, dusting, and cleaning. The task can be made easier by carefully going over your home, room by room, with an eye to eliminating as many "allergen traps" as possible. Many people are surprised to learn just how many hidden havens for allergens there are, even in relatively spartan rooms. Dr. John C. Selner, Clinical Professor of Pediatrics at the University of Colorado Health Sciences Center, recently published a detailed questionnaire in *The Journal of Respiratory Diseases* (January, 1986), in which he listed the types of questions that should be asked in assessing a home for asthma-triggering factors. These include:

Exterior

- What type of area do you live in? (urban, suburban, rural, etc.)

- Do you live near a street or road?

- Are there any nearby industrial complexes? Do you feel worse when you are near that site or when the wind is blowing from that direction?

- Does the house have a basement? Is there an adjoining or nearby garage? Are your symptoms worse when you are in either of these places?

- Has the house been remodeled recently? What type of insulation does it have? Has it been painted recently? Did your symptoms seem to be related to any of these changes?

- Do you feel worse when you come home?

- What kinds of trees, grasses, and other plants surround the house? Are any of these sprayed? If so, with what? Do you feel worse when working or playing in the yard?

- Do you use gas-powered tools, such as a lawn mower?

- Do you have a swimming pool? Is it in or near the

house? What kinds of chemicals are used in it? Is there a nearby pond or other source of standing water?

Interior

- What kind of heating system do you have (electric, gas, coal, wood, etc.)? Are the furnace air vents and ducts vacuumed or cleaned periodically? Do you have a working fireplace? What do you burn in it? Are your symptoms worse immediately after a fuel delivery?

- Do you notice an odor from mold or mildew in the bathrooms, basement, or other rooms?

- Are the walls papered? What kind of covering and adhesive were used? Is there mold or mildew growing under the paper?

- What kind of floor coverings do you have? If there are rugs, what type do you have (i.e., shag, flat weave, wall-to-wall, area, etc.)? What are they made from (i.e., wool, synthetics, straw, cotton, etc.)? How old are the rugs?

- Do you have upholstered furniture? What is it stuffed with (i.e., synthetics, kapok, flax or cottonseed, down, horsehair, rubber, etc.)? Do your symptoms seem worse when you are in a particular room or sitting on a certain chair or couch?

- What are your mattresses and pillows stuffed with (cotton, foam rubber, synthetics, feathers, etc.)?

- What kind of window coverings do you have (slat blinds, curtains, drapes, shades, etc.)? What are they made of? How often are they cleaned?

- What kinds of cleaners do you use (powders, sprays, ammonia or other chemical cleaners, detergents, polishes, waxes, etc.)? Is most of the cleaning done by sweeping? Dusting? Vacuuming? Washing? How often? Are symptoms better or worse following cleaning?

- Do you have air-conditioning? If so, what type (central, room, etc.)? Do you use a humidifier? Dehumidifier? Are these checked and cleaned periodically?

- What kind of cooking stove do you use (gas, electric, wood)? Do you have any gas appliances (refrigerator, clothes washer or dryer, water heater, freezer, etc.)? How old are your major appliances? Does the refrigerator have a drip tray? Is it emptied and cleaned regularly?

- Are there insects or rodents in the house? Do you use pesticides? What kinds?

- Are there any furry or feathered pets in the house? Did previous owners have a cat or other pet? If so, have rugs, drapes, upholstered furniture, etc., been changed?

- Do you have houseplants? If so, what kind?

- Do you use room fresheners? If so, what kind (sprays, solid stick, impregnated plastics or woods, incense, etc.)?

- Are there smokers in the household? Are symptoms worse when someone is smoking or soon thereafter, or in the presence of the smoker?

- Are the symptoms worse in a particular room, or in the presence of a certain person? Does he or she use scented soaps or cosmetics?

These are but a few of the many questions that should be considered in tracking down environmental substances that may worsen asthma. By studying the answers to this questionnaire, a specialist in environmental medicine or an allergist can help pinpoint possible hidden triggering factors that should be investigated further. For example, the filters on room air conditioners, humidifiers, or heating units can be checked for molds, microorganisms, and dust. A gas range may be exchanged for an electric one. The process can be tedious, and even going through each room from top to bottom may not uncover the offending objects. Recently, there has been a good deal of controversy surrounding the types of materials used in insulation and building materials. The solvents used in plywood and particle board and the chemicals used in insulating material are common examples of building materials that may provoke asthma symptoms.

Most people associate air pollution with smog and industrial chemicals. However, recent studies have found that the air inside homes and places of business may actually contain more pollutants than the air outdoors. Efforts to conserve energy by making buildings—both homes and offices—more airtight has, in some instances, added to the problem of indoor pollution. The airtight environment does not allow for as rapid exchange of air, and the recirculation of stale air exacerbates the problem. The air-conditioning and ventilation systems in these sealed buildings are often inadequate, and also provide an ideal growing place for bacteria, molds, and other organic allergens. Mobile homes or trailers tend to be particularly airtight, and often lack adequate ventilation for things like gas stoves or heating systems. They also may emit large amounts of solvents and other chemicals used in the building materials and insulation.

Although there is no doubt that excessive amounts of formaldehyde and other environmental chemicals can provoke asthma, it would be folly to assume that these ubiquitous substances are common triggers of asthma attacks. Caution and common sense must be used in tracking down and eliminating possible environmental allergens and irritants. In recent years, "environmental medicine" has become increas-

ingly popular, and there is considerable justification in looking for and correcting environmental causes of disease. Many
physicians who treat asthma, for example, will order an environmental survey of the patient's home or workplace and, in
the process, uncover hidden triggering factors. But the science often is imprecise and the good is sometimes overshad-
owed by misconceptions and even outright quackery. In dealing with any difficult chronic disease that has no cure, large
numbers of people will turn to questionable therapies, often
out of frustration or desperation. Before undertaking an expensive "environmental medicine" survey of your home or
undergoing extensive allergy-testing, check out the creden-
tials of the company or practitioner. Dr. Selner describes the
case of a woman who was living out of a car in the dead of
winter in Colorado after "tests" at an ecology medicine center in Chicago convinced her that braving the risk of freezing
to death outdoors was preferable to exposing herself to indoor pollutants.

Just how far one goes in trying to eliminate indoor pollutants depends upon many factors, including the severity of
the asthma, the clarity of its link to these environmental factors, and the complexity or ease of removing them. Solutions
may range from something as simple as removing or ex-
changing rugs and stuffed furniture, to moving out of the
house altogether and into one with a more controlled environment. Studies have found that in extreme cases, living in
an environment in which the building materials are primarily
stone or glass—substances that do not readily emit gases or
shed particles that can be inhaled—and one that can be carefully controlled for molds, dust and other inhalants, may result in dramatic improvement of asthma. But living in a glass
house or completely controlled environment is not easy, or
necessary, for the vast majority of asthmatic patients. Less
drastic commonsense measures usually will suffice. Following
are suggestions frequently put forth at National Jewish.

Avoid using aerosol sprays. This includes a long list of common products, such as hair sprays, oven cleaners, deodorants, air fresheners, and pesticides, among others. It is impossible to avoid breathing in sprayed products that linger in the air, and these products contain propellants and other ingredients that affect hyperreactive airways.

Check air-conditioning and heating units. Make sure that filters in these units are changed or cleaned regularly. Avoid window fans, which tend to draw pollen, molds and other airborne irritants into the house. Air conditioners should be of the type that recirculates the air, rather than the type that draws in air from the outside and cools it (often with its own chemical irritant), and then blows it into the room.

Do not keep pets in the home. Pets play an important part in many people's lives, and this is perhaps the most difficult sacrifice for many asthmatics. Parting with a beloved dog, cat, parrot, or other furry or feathered pet is hard, especially when the animal does not seem to provoke symptoms. Still, asthma experts, including the physicians at National Jewish, stress that animal dander, saliva, and urine all are potent airway allergens, and that even if a person does not suffer immediate symptoms, the presence of these animals in a household makes asthma control much more difficult. Many myths abound regarding the safety of some pets versus others. For example, many people have the mistaken notion that a Rex cat, which does not shed, or a poodle that is clipped frequently, are acceptable. Others think that a caged animal, such as a gerbil or rabbit, will not pose a problem. However, these animals still shed dander and produce saliva and urine that are potent allergens. In short, there are no nonallergenic cats, dogs, or furry animals. Some people compromise by keeping reptiles or interesting home aquariums—an acceptable alternative so long as the water is properly circulated and changed frequently to prevent growth of molds, bacteria, and other microorganisms.

Ban all smoking in the house. From the asthmatic's point of view, it would be better to ban all smoking, period. Since this is not realistic, at least the patient's home environment can be kept free of tobacco smoke. People who are especially sensitive to tobacco may encounter problems simply in being around a smoker, since the fumes and pollutants cling to the smoker's hair and clothes. Certainly, no asthmatic should smoke; and all members of the household should make every effort not to smoke themselves, even if they do not have asthma. Dr. Mason repeatedly stresses that "all asthmatics deserve a smoke-free environment called home!" (See Chapter 9 on *Smoking and Asthma* for a more detailed discussion.)

Prevent air from becoming too dry. Dry air contains more dust and other inhalants than more humid air, and thus a humidifier may be an important piece of home equipment for the asthmatic. There are several types of room humidifiers available. Because the models that have a water reservoir system may harbor molds and bacteria, the types that emit an intermittent humidifying spray that is controlled by a thermostat are preferable. Humidifiers should be cleaned regularly with vinegar or dilute acetic acid to prevent growth of molds and other microorganisms.

Pay particular attention to the bedroom. If possible, try to create a controlled "oasis" where the asthmatic sleeps or spends a good deal of time. If need be, a circulating room air conditioner and baseboard electric heating unit can be installed in this room to help seal it from the rest of the house. Mattresses and pillows should be covered with a plastic material that has been aired until it no longer smells. Obviously, down, feathers, kapok, and other highly allergenic substances should be eliminated from this room. Draperies, curtains, rugs, and other dust-catchers also should be avoided. The room should be vacuumed regularly, and bedding should be washed every few days. Make sure the laundered items are thoroughly rinsed, and avoid any detergents that provoke symptoms. Stuffed toys and live animals should be kept out of an asthmatic child's room.

Make sure all gas and oil appliances and kitchen ranges are well ventilated. Appliances can be a major source of airway irritants for asthma patients. Things like kerosene heaters should be avoided, and gas or oil-burning furnaces and stoves should be well ventilated with efficient filtering systems. The kitchen range is a major source of fumes and irritants. An electric range should be used instead of gas or wood. The ordinary range hood usually is not efficient enough to filter out fumes produced by cooking. Investing in a laboratory-type hood exhaust system for the kitchen range may be advisable, especially if a patient's asthma is poorly controlled and worsened by exposure to kitchen fumes.

Avoid furniture dust traps. Items like wall-to-wall carpeting, shag rugs, and furniture upholstered with kapok, horsehair, and other allergy-producing substances, all should be avoided. Rugs are notorious. They can harbor huge numbers of dust mites, and vacuuming stirs up both dust and mites. If rugs cannot be avoided, select area rugs that are tightly woven and can be washed. Tiles are an ideal floor covering because they do not collect dust or give off gases. Plain wood is also a good covering; vinyl and other floor covering may give off small amounts of petroleum gases, but the amount is so small that if the covering is aired until there is no longer a smell, they usually can be tolerated.

Seal off garage area from the house, especially the bedroom. Fumes from fuels are common asthma triggers, and bedrooms located adjacent to garage areas can be a problem for asthmatics. If possible, the garage and bedrooms should be separated, and the garage tightly sealed from the rest of the house so that its fumes do not invade living areas.

Avoid chemical cleaners that may provoke asthma. The problem with aerosol cleaners was discussed earlier; a number of other household cleaners also may contain airway irritants. Products that contain petrochemicals or substances like ammonia, pine oil, ethylenediamine, chlorophenols, or organic solvents are common offenders. If symptoms worsen when using a particular cleaner, or on the heels of general housecleaning, try switching to other cleaning products. Baking soda, chlorine bleaches, soap, mineral or lemon oil furniture polish, and vinegar are common examples of cleaners that do not contain petrochemicals or ammonia.

Consider an air-purifying device. There are a large number of air filters and purifying devices on the market; some asthmatics insist they provide relief but many others do not, and it is a good idea to seek professional guidance before investing in a particular model or system. The function of an air purifier is to filter out as many pollutants and particles, such as dust and pollen, as possible. In general, an air purifier should recirculate the air at least four times per hour. The types of air filters generally recommended are (1) the high-efficiency particulate-arresting devices, which have a very fine screen to trap even very tiny particles; and (2) electrostatic or ionizing devices that draw particles to an electrostatically charged filter. There also are a variety of fiber filters. Charcoal filters will trap things like tobacco smoke, but generally are not efficient enough to serve as adequate air purifiers. All air-purifying devices have filters that need periodic cleaning or replacement. Some are noisy and some may produce their own pollutants. The electrostatic devices, for example, produce ozone, which in itself is an irritant for many people. Ionizing devices can handle only relatively small areas, so several may be needed. It is a good idea to rent a particular unit before actually buying it to make sure it is what you need.

Dealing with the Outside Environment

Of course, very few people, including even severe asthmatics, spend all of their time in a controlled home environment. It is one thing to control the indoor environment and quite another to cope with what goes on in the world at large. Not uncommonly, a person will be fine at home, but will begin to wheeze when at school, the workplace, the supermarket, in the car, or even simply when outdoors. Detective work, similar to that used to identify asthma triggers in the home, usually can help pinpoint specific allergens or irritants in those places in which the person with asthma must spend considerable time. The best tool for this detective work is a peak-flow meter. Once the triggering factors are identified, most asthmatics can manage quite well by avoiding these factors whenever possible, and using medication or desensitization to minimize the effects of whatever factors cannot be avoided.

Prudence and common sense can go a long way toward minimizing the effects of environmental triggering factors. For example, during periods of cold, wind, and high pollution, such as a smog alert, people with asthma and other lung disorders often are advised to stay indoors as much as possible. People who suffer only during the fall ragweed season, for example, may be able to arrange their lives so that they can avoid exposure; some who can afford the time and expense simply pack up and move to the seashore or some other place that is free of ragweed at this time. Preventive medication can be used prior to anticipated exposure to known triggering factors. For example, a child who is particularly sensitive to animal dander, but is determined to join an outing to the circus or zoo, often can do so if the proper medication is used in advance. (The special problems of workplace-induced asthma are discussed in Chapter 13.)

Without a doubt, a person who must deal with a long list of environmental asthma triggers can find it to be time-consuming, frustrating, and sometimes restricting and discouraging. Asthma is not an easy disease; on the brighter side, it should be stressed that for most patients, the triggering factors can be identified and the asthma controlled. In the uncovering of environmental factors, the emphasis should be on objective data, such as readings from the peak flow meter, whenever possible, rather than vague symptoms.

CHAPTER 8

Other Conditions That Worsen Asthma

In the previous chapter, we concentrated on the relationship between allergies and asthma. Whereas allergies may be the most familiar condition affecting asthma, they are by no means alone. There are other, often overlooked conditions that can aggravate asthma, and controlling these frequently results in a marked improvement of overall asthma management.

The Nose and Sinuses

The nose and nasal passage are designed to moisten, warm, and cleanse the air before it moves into the lower respiratory tract. In addition to being the uppermost part of the respiratory system, the nose is also intricately associated with the sinuses and inner parts of the ear. The sinuses are hollow spaces located behind and above the nose. There are four sets of sinuses, which are connected by a series of narrow openings. The sinuses are lined with mucus-producing tissue; their major function is to drain and cleanse facial and nasal tissue and to produce mucus for the nose. The hollow spaces also lighten the skull and are important in the production of sound.

Postnasal drip, which is drainage of mucus from the nasal passages and sinuses into the back of the throat, can get into the lungs, especially when a person is sleeping. During the day the larynx prevents the mucus from entering the airways, but during sleep the larynx relaxes and the mucus can enter the lung. This drainage can trigger bronchospasms and lead to an asthma attack. In fact, National Jewish studies have documented that nasal drainage can be a major cause of nocturnal asthma, attacks that come on for no apparent reason during sleep.

Patients at National Jewish are taught how to do nasal washings—an important self-care measure intended to keep the nose clean and open and to reduce nasal swelling. (See Table 8 on *How to Do Nasal Washes.*)

The sinus openings are narrow and can easily become blocked by mucus and other debris. When this happens, the sinuses themselves also may become clogged and inflamed, a condition called *sinusitis.* An uncomfortable, congested feeling, headaches, swelling around the eyes, and, in severe cases, fever and a pus-filled nasal discharge are common symptoms of sinusitis. Asthmatics seem to be more vulnerable to sinusitis than is the general population; many have chronic sinusitis without even knowing it. Although sinusitis does not cause asthma, it can lead to more frequent attacks and make the disease more difficult to control.

X rays of the sinuses will confirm a diagnosis of sinusitis, as well as detect asymptomatic swollen tissue, blocked passages, and the presence of fluid in the hollow spaces. Sinusitis can be difficult to treat, especially if it is a long-standing condition. Antibiotic therapy, usually for four to six weeks and often even longer, may be prescribed. Sinus washes or irrigation also may be needed to reduce swelling and to clear out mucus, bacteria, dead cells, and other debris. Decongestants, antihistamines, and topical steroids also may be prescribed,

Table 8
How to Do Nasal Washes

Nasal washes are intended to keep the nasal passages open, reduce swelling and remove bacteria and mucus. A warm saline solution—one-fourth to one-half teaspoon of salt in a glass of warm water—is used. Care should be taken that the salt solution is not too weak or too strong, as either extreme can irritate the nasal passages. One of two methods can be used:

Method One

1. Pour some of the saline solution into the palm of your hand or a small shallow medicine cup.

2. With head bent far over sink, pinch one nostril closed with your finger and "sniff" the liquid up your nose, one nostril at a time. The sniffing will draw the salt water through the nostril into the back of the throat. This may produce coughing, which will bring up accumulated mucus.

3. Spit the liquid out through your mouth. Blow your nose lightly afterward. Repeat until the only material coughed up or blown from the nose is the salt solution.

Method Two

1. Fill a large, all-rubber ear syringe, which can be purchased at any drugstore, with saline solution.

2. Lean over a sink with your head down. Pinch one nostril closed with a finger and insert syringe tip just inside the other nostril. Pinch around the syringe tip to keep solution from running out of your nose. Gently squeeze the syringe and release the bulb several times to swish the solution around the nose; then squeeze the bulb hard enough to force saline up over the palate in the roof of the mouth. Spit it out and repeat for the other nostril. As with Method One, accumulated mucus should be coughed up and spit out.

but these should be used only upon a doctor's specific recommendation. Many people with nasal and sinus congestion resort to nonprescription nasal sprays like Afrin or Neosynephrine to unclog nasal and sinus passages. Brief use of these sprays for a day or two during a cold may not cause harm, but many people—especially asthmatics—with chronic sinusitis end up using them continuously, sometimes every two or three hours, day in and day out for years. As time goes by, increasingly frequent doses of the sprays are needed to keep the nasal passages clear. Overuse of the sprays can lead to swelling of the sinuses and nasal passages from the medication itself, a condition referred to as *rhinitis medicamentosa*.

Ear Infections

Babies and young children are particularly vulnerable to ear infections, and youngsters with asthma and/or hay fever seem to have an even higher than normal incidence of ear problems. In young children, the Eustachian tube, which connects the nose and the ear, is very narrow and is easily blocked by only a small amount of mucus or other secretions. This provides an ideal place for bacteria to thrive, leading to infection.

Antibiotics usually can clear up the infection, but many youngsters, especially those with asthma, are plagued with frequently recurrent ear infections. Since chronic or frequent ear infections can cause permanent hearing loss, the problem should not be ignored. Pain in the ears, fever, and other symptoms of infection should be seen to by a doctor without delay; and after a full course of antibiotic treatment, the child should be taken back to the doctor to check for remaining fluid and swelling in the ear. Sometimes special tubes need to be placed in the eardrum to promote the flow of air in the middle ear, and also to help reduce the likelihood of infection by augmenting the Eustachian tube's drainage capacity.

Esophageal Reflux

The esophagus is the tube that carries food from the mouth to the stomach. Normally, the esophageal sphincter—a smooth muscle that joins the esophagus and stomach—prevents digestive acids and other stomach contents from flowing back into the esophagus. Some of the medications prescribed to treat asthma work by relaxing smooth muscles in the airways; these same drugs also relax other smooth muscles, including the esophageal sphincter. When a person is in an upright position, gravity helps prevent a backflow, or reflux, of stomach contents into the esophagus; however, problems may occur when lying down. People with esophageal reflux often awaken at night with heartburn. Heartburn can produce chest pains that radiate to the jaw, shoulders, or back. Not uncommonly, a person with heartburn will fear that he or she is having a heart attack; similarly, people who are having a heart attack often dismiss it as an attack of heartburn.

Asthmatics with esophageal reflux often awaken with wheezing and other symptoms during the night. They also may notice a bitter or sour taste in the mouth, an indication that stomach juices have backed up along the entire length of the esophagus. Some of these acids may enter the trachea and then flow into the respiratory system. The resulting irritation can produce the bronchoconstriction characteristic of an asthma attack. Any asthma patient who suffers nighttime attacks should consider esophageal reflux as a possible triggering factor.

Reflux can be confirmed by several tests. The most common is a biologic assay in which a small probe is inserted into the esophagus and left for twelve to sixteen hours. This measures the acidity in the esophagus. A pH level below 5.0 for five minutes indicates reflux. A peak-flow meter can confirm the effects on the lungs. The esophagus also may be tested for inflammation (the Bernstein test), an indication of reflux. In the Bernstein test, either acid or saline is infused into the esophagus through a nasogastric tube, and symptoms and pulmonary functions are recorded.

The effects of esophageal reflux can be minimized by avoiding lying down for a couple of hours after eating and avoiding foods that cause heartburn or excessive acid production, such as coffee, tea, and other sources of caffeine; spicy foods, and nuts and other fatty foods. Antacids also help reduce stomach acids, and of course anyone with heartburn problems should avoid smoking. In addition to these commonsense measures, patients troubled by esophageal reflux are advised to elevate the head of the bed six to eight inches. This can be done by placing a wooden block or stack of thick books or other hard objects under the headboard to raise the top of the bed so that it is higher than the foot of the bed. Pillows or wedges placed under the mattress should be avoided since these may cause the sleeper to bend at the waist, a position that promotes reflux.

Bronchopulmonary Aspergillosis

Some asthmatics develop a condition called bronchiectasis, characterized by widening and irregularity of the larger air tubes in the lungs and increased mucus production. These patients are vulnerable to aspergillosis, a chronic lung condition in which *Aspergillus* fungus grows along the airways. Patients become allergic to the fungus and then develop local inflammation in the airtubes, which exacerbates their asthma and bronchiectasis. This condition can be diagnosed through antibody and skin tests. Other fungi can grow in the lungs, but *Aspergillus* is the most common.

Although fungal infections of the airway are relatively rare, the possibility should be considered when asthma becomes more resistant to treatment. There also may be changes in the mucus; patients often report that their cough is more severe and persistent, and the mucus produced is thicker or more discolored than before. After a diagnosis of bronchopulmonary aspergillosis has been confirmed, the fungus usually can be eradicated by drugs, especially steroids, to control the asthma and inflammation and to allow the body's natural defenses to clear out the fungus.

The Menstrual Cycle

Some women experience a worsening of their asthma during the premenstrual phase of their monthly cycles. The reasons for this are unknown, although researchers believe hormonal changes may play a role. A possible association with the menstrual cycle can be documented by having the woman keep a careful diary of symptoms and relating this to menstruation. A woman who finds that she invariably experiences increased attacks in the week before her period can increase her medication at this time to either prevent or minimize the symptoms. As with other premenstrual symptoms, the use of nonsteroidal anti-inflammatory drugs, such as ibuprofen, may help. But before these drugs are used, the woman should make sure that she is not sensitive to them. For example, patients whose asthma is worsened by aspirin often find the same sensitivity to nonsteroidal anti-inflammatory agents.

CHAPTER 9
Smoking and Asthma

By now, everyone knows that smoking is one of the worst things anyone can do to his or her lungs. According to the Surgeon General of the United States, smoking is responsible for some 350,000 deaths in this country each year, approximately six times the total United States deaths in the war in Vietnam. It is the major cause of lung cancer, emphysema, chronic bronchitis, and other respiratory disorders. In fact, more than 85 percent of all lung cancer victims have smoked and, in general, smokers have twice as many respiratory illnesses as nonsmokers. Smoking also increases the risk of a heart attack—the Surgeon General estimates that more than 225,000 heart attack deaths each year are linked to smoking. And it should come as no surprise that smoking, both active and passive, is particularly harmful to asthmatics.

Most asthmatics are well aware of the fact that tobacco smoke makes their asthma worse. Simply being around someone who smokes will often produce wheezing and other symptoms. Indeed, tobacco smoke is a common inhaled asthma-triggering factor. Tobacco smoke works in several ways to worsen asthma:

- Tobacco smoke contains a number of irritants that increase the airways' protective bronchospasm, a response that is a potent asthma-triggering factor.

- Smoking damages the cilia, the tiny hair-like structures of the lung that keep the airways clear of mucus. This results in delayed clearance of inhaled particles and thus an added buildup of sticky mucus to clog the airways and promote infection.

- Tobacco smoke contains more than four thousand different components, including carbon monoxide and a dozen or so other gases; tar and other irritating particulates; nicotine, a powerful stimulant and addictive agent; foreign substances, such as pesticides; and poisons like cyanide and arsenic. Many of the components in tobacco and its smoke irritate the airways, producing a chronic (smoker's) cough and increased mucus secretion, all of which worsen asthma. In addition, many of the natural and added components of tobacco and tobacco smoke are irritants that trigger asthma.

- Smoking impairs the body's ability to clear inhaled microorganisms, thereby increasing the likelihood of infection.

- Smoking increases the level of carbon monoxide in the body and lowers the amount of oxygen transported to cells via the circulation. This can be particularly serious to asthmatics with coronary heart disease, who already may have reduced oxygen and increased carbon monoxide.

- Smoking constricts small blood vessels, causing an immediate rise in the heart rate and blood pressure.

- Smoking causes emphysema and chronic bronchitis, conditions that worsen the effects of asthma.

- Smoking interferes with the action of several important asthma medications. For example, it causes the body to use theophylline much faster than normal. Larger doses of the drug may be needed to overcome asthma symptoms, which are made worse by the smoking. Higher drug dosages increase the risk of side effects, and to control the asthma an additional medication, such as a corticosteroid, may be needed. Long-term use of steroids carries a higher risk of serious drug side effects (see Chapter 16).

- Smoking increases the incidence of stomach ulcers, and also encourages the backflow of stomach juices into the esophagus (esophageal reflux). If these gastric acids reach the mouth—as often happens when reflux occurs while sleeping—some may enter the windpipe and flow into the airways, causing irritation and constriction, and triggering an attack of asthma. (See Chapter 8.)

Obviously, anyone with asthma or any other lung disorder should make every effort to stop smoking. But tobacco smoke can be a major problem even for nonsmokers with asthma; for these individuals, passive smoking—breathing in the smoke from other people's cigarettes, cigars, or pipes—can be almost as harmful as active smoking. Two thirds of the smoke produced by a cigarette goes into the environment. Indoor pollution from cigarettes can far exceed the safety standards set for outdoor pollution. It is only recently that the tremendous health hazards of passive smoking have come to light. For example, Dr. C. Everett Koop, the Surgeon General of the United States, estimates that 5,000 Americans die each year from passive smoking. The hazards of maternal smoking on the fetus and newborn infant are well known—low birth weight, miscarriages, stillbirths, and crib death all are more common in families with mothers who smoke. Babies of parents who smoke have more than twice the incidence of pneumonia and bronchitis during the first year of life. Studies also have found that young children of parents who smoke have twice as many respiratory problems as children whose parents do not smoke. Children exposed to second-hand smoke in a small room for thirty minutes have increased heart rate, higher blood pressure, and a rise in the carbon monoxide level of their blood. Parents of children with asthma should definitely not smoke.

Children are by no means the only sufferers of second-hand smoke. Studies have found that nonsmokers who are exposed to tobacco smoke at work for many years have reduced lung function and increased lung and nasal symptoms. Spouses of heavy smokers have a higher than normal incidence of lung cancer. Employers are increasingly aware of the health hazards of passive smoking, especially since some workers have been awarded disability benefits and worker's compensation because of workplace exposure to tobacco smoke. A number of Federal agencies, as well as states and localities, also have passed laws mandating that employees have a smoke-free work environment if they so desire.

Smoking Cessation

Doctors at National Jewish stress that it is absolutely vital that asthmatic patients not smoke, and that all asthmatics should have as smoke-free an environment as possible. Since we live in a society in which some 30 million people smoke, it is obviously very difficult—if not impossible—to eliminate *all* exposure to tobacco smoke. Simply entering many public places such as restaurants, hotel lobbies, and office buildings, and even the private homes of friends, usually entails exposure to varying amounts of tobacco smoke. But at the very least, an asthmatic's own home should be off-limits to all smoking; and, if possible, the workplace should also be as smoke-free as possible. Parents and spouses of asthma patients must realize the importance of a smoke-free environment. "If family members really care about the patient, they will not permit any smoking in the house," Dr. Mason stresses.

Smoking cessation is an important part of the treatment program at National Jewish. Any asthma patient who smokes will certainly be persuaded to stop, as part of his or her asthma-control program. Not uncommonly, an asthmatic may live in a household where someone else smokes. A child, for example, may have one or both parents who smoke; or an adult may have a spouse or roommate who smokes. "We explain to these family members how important their not smoking is in our joint efforts to bring a patient's asthma under control," says Dr. Reuben M. Cherniack. "Very often, persuading—and helping—parents or spouses to stop smoking is a key to bringing a patient's asthma under control."

No one disputes the health benefits of not smoking, but actually stopping is often very difficult. Nicotine is a powerful addictive substance, and once a person is hooked on tobacco, it is very difficult to stop. And there are certain groups for whom stopping is particularly difficult. For example, studies have found that women often have more difficulty in stopping than men. The more cigarettes per day a person smokes, the harder it is to quit. Smokers who started at an early age and smoke two or more packs a day encounter more problems in stopping than people who took up the habit as adults and who smoke a pack or less a day.

Instead of quitting, many smokers switch to filter or low-tar, low-nicotine cigarettes in the mistaken belief that these are somehow "safe." Although there is some evidence that these products may carry a slightly lower risk of cancer than regular cigarettes, they are by no means safe; they still are very irritating to the lungs, and there is some evidence that filtered cigarettes actually increase the risk of heart disease. The smoke still contains a toxic amount of carbon monoxide and other harmful substances. In addition, studies of smoking habits have found that people who switch to low-tar, low-nicotine brands often end up smoking more, not less; and that in the end they take in as much of these harmful ingredients as when they smoked regular cigarettes.

Many smokers, including patients with asthma, emphysema, and other serious lung disorders, rationalize their continued smoking by saying, "I've smoked all these years, and the damage is done. Why stop now?" This, too, is a false assumption; doctors at National Jewish stress that no matter how long a patient has smoked or how serious the lung condition, he or she can benefit from stopping. Instructors in the smoking cessation program repeatedly emphasize that "It is not too late. Stopping smoking can do you considerable good, no matter how severe your lung disease. It is more than worth the bother!"

National Jewish doctors recognize that their patients may have extra difficulty in giving up smoking. "Chronic illnesses, such as asthma, increase stress," Dr. Cherniack explains, "and stress makes it more difficult to break a habit, such as smoking. Many of our patients insist that they smoke because it calms them down and relieves stress." In reality, smoking does the opposite because it worsens their lung condition, which adds to the stress. And while smokers may think that a cigarette calms jittery nerves, it actually adds to nervous tension by prompting the body to increase secretion of epinephrine, one of the stress hormones that instigate the body's fight-or-flight response. This is what causes the heart to beat faster and the blood pressure to rise, and produces the other immediate effects of smoking, such as a sudden surge of energy, or "smoker's high."

Strategies for Stopping Smoking

There are many strategies for stopping smoking, and what works well for one person may not necessarily be the best approach for another. It is estimated that about 33 million Americans have stopped smoking since the first Surgeon General's report on smoking and health came out in 1964. Studies have found that most of these ex-smokers did not succeed in quitting on the first try; at least 70 percent of the people who have successfully given up smoking attempted to stop at least once before they finally managed to quit for good. Some studies have put the relapse rate as high as 90 percent. Each successive try, however, is likely to produce some permanent success. Thus, doctors stress that if you do not succeed in stopping the first time around, don't be discouraged; simply try again and again, if need be, until you no longer smoke.

Ninety to 95 percent of those who stop smoking succeed in stopping on their own, and quitting "cold turkey" seems to produce the best results. For those who cannot tolerate stopping all at once, a gradual reduction in the number of cigarettes smoked each day may work. Practicing self-hypnosis has produced good results for some people. Dr. Herbert Spiegel, a psychiatrist at Columbia University's College of Physicians and Surgeons, has taught self-hypnosis to more than 10,000 patients who want to stop smoking. Most of these patients came to Dr. Spiegel as a last resort—they had tried stopping before and had used numerous other techniques. Long-term follow-up of these patients has found that nearly two thirds managed to stop permanently by using self-hypnosis, and that certain subsets of patients—for example, people who were easily hypnotized and those who lived with a spouse or partner—had a success rate of 90 percent or better.

Chewing nicotine-containing gum has been a boon to some smokers who are heavily addicted to nicotine. Doctors at National Jewish suggest this as an aid to smokers who are having nicotine-withdrawal problems. However, the gum should be used for only a few weeks, as it, too, can be habit-forming and exert many of the harmful cardiovascular effects of nicotine. Still, this is not as big a health hazard as continued smoking. National Jewish patients are advised that the important function of nicotine gum is to help the smoker break the smoking habit in two stages: First comes the actual smoking cessation, and elimination of the ritual aspects of smoking such as the handling of cigarettes, the actual inhaling, and other pleasurable aspects associated with smoking. Second, after a person has become accustomed to not smoking, he or she can then deal with eliminating the nicotine addiction. It takes only about forty-eight hours to rid the body entirely of nicotine, so for most people the withdrawal period is quite manageable.

Tips for Planning to Stop Smoking

Every smoker is different, so self-analysis and advance planning are important in increasing the chances of success. The accompanying self-assessment quiz, developed by the National Clearinghouse for Smoking and Health, can be used to pinpoint why a person smokes and to hone in on the most appropriate strategies for that person to use in order to stop. Following are specific tips that have been helpful to others.

Table 9
Why Do You Smoke? A Self-Assessment Quiz

Following are statements people use to describe what they derive from smoking. Rate how these statements apply to you according to this scale:

5 = always	3 = occasionally	1 = never
4 = frequently	2 = seldom	

A. I smoke cigarettes in order to keep myself from slowing down. _____

B. Handling a cigarette is part of the enjoyment of smoking. _____

C. Smoking cigarettes is pleasant and relaxing. _____

D. I light up a cigarette when I feel angry about something. _____

E. When I run out of cigarettes, I find it almost unbearable until I can get more. _____

F. I smoke cigarettes automatically without even being aware of it. _____

G. I smoke cigarettes to stimulate me, to perk myself up. _____

H. Part of the enjoyment of smoking comes from the steps I take to light up. _____

I. I find cigarettes pleasurable. _____

J. When I feel uncomfortable or upset about something, I light up a cigarette. _____

K. I am very much aware of the fact when I am not smoking a cigarette. _____

L. I light up a cigarette without realizing I still have one burning in the ashtray. _____

M. I smoke cigarettes to give me a "lift." _____

N. When I smoke a cigarette, part of the enjoyment is watching the smoke as I exhale it. _____

O. I want a cigarette most when I am comfortable and relaxed. _____

P. When I feel "blue" or want to take my mind off cares and worries, I smoke cigarettes. _____

Q. I get a real gnawing for a cigarette when I haven't smoked one for a while. _____

R. I've found a cigarette in my mouth and didn't remember putting it there. _____

How to Score:

1. Enter the numbers you have selected for the test questions in the space below, putting the number you have selected for question A over line A, for question B over line B, etc.

2. Total the three scores on each line to get your totals. For example, the sum of scores over lines A, G, and M gives you your score on Stimulation. Scores of 11 or more for a category indicate that this factor is an important source of satisfaction. Scores of 7 or less are low and

probably indicate that this factor does not apply to you. Scores in between are marginal.

_____	+	_____	+	_____	=	_____
(A)		(G)		(M)		Stimulation
_____	+	_____	+	_____	=	_____
(B)		(H)		(N)		Handling
_____	+	_____	+	_____	=	_____
(C)		(I)		(O)		Relaxation
_____	+	_____	+	_____	=	_____
(D)		(J)		(P)		Crutch
_____	+	_____	+	_____	=	_____
(E)		(K)		(Q)		Craving
_____	+	_____	+	_____	=	_____
(F)		(L)		(R)		Habit

Interpreting Your Score:

Stimulation: You smoke because it gives you a lift. Try substituting a brisk walk or a few simple exercises.

Handling: You like the ritual and trappings of smoking. Find other ways to keep your hands busy. Knitting, doodling, even twiddling your thumbs are possibilities.

Relaxation: You get a real sense of pleasure out of smoking. An honest consideration of the harmful effects may remove the pleasure.

Crutch: If you smoke mostly when you are angry or depressed, you may be using cigarettes as a tranquilizer. In a difficult situation, take a deep breath to relax, or call a friend to talk over your feelings. Learning new coping strategies to substitute for smoking will help greatly in quitting.

Craving: Quitting smoking may be more difficult if you are psychologically or physiologically dependent, but once you have stopped, it will be possible to resist the temptation to smoke because the withdrawal effort is too much to go through again.

Habit: If you smoke without even realizing you are doing so, it should be relatively easy to break the habit. Start by asking, "Do I really want this cigarette?" Change smoking patterns and make cigarettes more difficult to get.

(Self-test adapted from *Smoker's Self Test* by Daniel Horn, Ph.D., Director of the National Clearinghouse for Smoking and Health, U.S. Public Health Service. *Interpreting Your Score* adapted from "7-Day Plan to Help You Stop Smoking Cigarettes," The American Cancer Society, New York, 1978.)

List the reasons why you want to stop smoking. Some of the more common are outlined in Table 10, *Reasons to Quit Smoking.* You undoubtedly can add many more to the list.

Table 10

Reasons to Quit Smoking

---

1. Stopping will add years to your life.

2. Stopping will help avoid lung cancer, emphysema, bronchitis, heart attacks, and other serious illnesses.

3. You will get rid of your smoker's cough.

4. Stopping will increase stamina and endurance.

5. You will regain your sense of smell and of taste.

6. Your hair and clothes will not smell of stale tobacco.

7. Smoking increases facial wrinkling of women, making them look years older.

8. Stopping will help get rid of bad breath.

9. Stopping will save money, probably thousands of dollars each year.

10. Stopping will eliminate ugly stains on teeth and fingers.

11. Stopping will make you more pleasant to have around.

12. Stopping will help eliminate a health hazard for others forced to breath your second-hand smoke.

13. You will stop burning holes in clothes and furniture.

14. Stopping will remove a common fire hazard threatening your home and the lives of loved ones.

15. Stopping will demonstrate your willpower and self-control.

16. _____ (fill in)

17. _____

18. _____

Keep a diary of your smoking habits. This is similar to the diary of symptoms that asthmatics are urged to keep to identify triggering factors. Note the time of day and the circumstances under which each cigarette is smoked. For example: 7:30 A.M., cigarette with morning coffee. This diary can be used to pinpoint the times when a person is most likely to want a cigarette, and to substitute other activities at such times. In addition, if a smoker finds that he or she always has a cigarette with coffee, ending a meal with tea or skipping the coffee and taking a short walk instead may help break the routine.

Start to get in shape physically. This is good for both the asthma and as an aid in stopping smoking. It is difficult, if not impossible, to smoke while peddling an exercise bicycle, swimming, or engaging in other physical activities. Plan an exercise session for periods of time when you often smoke. Exercise also contributes to feelings of control and well-being —important aids in stopping smoking.

Change to another brand of cigarette. Although there is no safe cigarette, especially for a person with asthma or another lung disorder, switching brands as part of a strategy for quitting may be helpful. A new brand may not "taste" as good or be as pleasurable to smoke, which may make giving up smoking seem like less of a sacrifice.

Make smoking inconvenient. Throw out all your ashtrays, buy only one pack at a time, and throw away all but a couple of cigarettes, so that reaching for one is not as easy. Try to spend as much time as possible in places where smoking is prohibited. Museums, movie theaters, nonsmoking sections of trains and other means of transportation, are examples of places where smoking is not allowed.

Focus on the unpleasant aspects of smoking. Collect all your cigarette butts in a jar for a week or so and keep it displayed in a prominent place to remind you of how unattractive smoking can be. Get your teeth cleaned and resolve not to let them become yellowed and stained again. Send your clothes to the cleaners and resolve to keep them smelling fresh. Gather up garments, furniture, and other objects that have been marred by cigarette burns and put them in a prominent place to remind you of the damage caused by smoking.

When You're Ready to Quit . . .

Set a date for stopping smoking. Pick a time when you are not likely to be under a lot of stress. For example, it is not a good idea to quit just at a time when you are taking a new job, moving, studying for examinations, and so on. A vacation time or the beginning of a long weekend may be good choices. Or if you like company, try the day of the American Cancer Society's annual Smokeout, when several million other people will be abstaining from cigarettes.

Get rid of all cigarettes and other smoking paraphernalia. Make sure you have no hidden cigarettes around the house or office. Remove all ashtrays, matches, lighters, and other reminders of smoking. Tell your friends and family members to refuse to lend you a cigarette, even when you ask.

Enlist the support of others. Let your family members, work or school associates, close friends, and anyone else who may be helpful know your plans. The more people who are encouraging and supportive of your efforts, the greater your chances of success.

Make plans for the money you will save by not smoking. Put a glass jar on your desk or dresser and at the end of each day, deposit in it the money you would normally have spent on cigarettes. Review insurance policies to determine whether your premium will be lowered by not smoking. Calculate how many days you miss from work and how much more you spend on medical bills because of your smoking. (The national average is $2,000 to $4,000, and for asthmatics, the medical costs of smoking may be much higher.) Add in the savings on cleaning bills, dental visits, and other often-over-looked indirect costs of smoking. Chances are that you will end up with several thousands of dollars that can be ear-marked for a vacation or some other substantial reward for not smoking.

Talk to your doctor. Your doctor has probably told you many times that you should stop smoking, but see if you can spend a few minutes going over your intentions with him or her. Studies have found that as little as five minutes of indi-vidual counselling from a doctor increases the likelihood of success in stopping smoking.

Know what to expect when you quit. Withdrawal symptoms rarely last for more than a couple of weeks, and for most people, the worst is over in the first two or three days. Surveys of former smokers have found that 40 to 50 percent experience no withdrawal symptoms. Others report a variety of symptoms, such as headaches, irritability, muscle aches, nervousness, or "feeling jittery." Some symptoms may be due to the body's healing process. For example, tingling sen-sations in the arms and legs may be a sign of improved circu-lation. Some people experience increased coughing in the first few days after stopping; this may be due to the lungs' clearing out the tar and other residue of smoking. Drinking plenty of water will help speed the clearance of nicotine from the body. The important thing is to recognize that these symptoms all are temporary, and that with each passing day there is less desire to smoke.

Pay attention to your diet. Almost immediately after people have stopped smoking, their senses of taste and smell begin to recover. Most smokers are amazed to find they had forgot-ten how good food can taste. Appetites improve and most people do gain a few pounds after stopping smoking. Indeed, many people use this anticipated weight gain as an excuse to continue smoking. Experts have estimated that the average person would have to gain seventy-five to one hundred pounds to offset the benefits of stopping smoking. Weight gain can be avoided by increasing exercise and eating filling but low-calorie foods, such as carrots and celery sticks, high-fiber crackers, plain popcorn, rice cakes, or fruit instead of things like peanuts, chips, candies, and other high-calorie, low-nutrient snack foods. Strive for a balanced diet, with about 60 percent of your calories coming from starches and other carbohydrates, 25 to 30 percent from fats, and 15 percent from protein. In the beginning, a little extra protein helps your body repair the damage from smoking. Avoid sugars, which promote swings in blood sugar and can worsen feelings of irritability and mood swings.

Keep alcohol consumption to a minimum. Many people smoke whenever they have a drink. Alcohol also lowers willpower, and increases the chance of a relapse.

Squelch your cigarette cravings. Study your smoking diary to determine the times and circumstances that seem to promote smoking for you. Plan alternative activities; try meditating or breathing exercises when you feel an urge to smoke. Call a supportive friend, take the dog for a walk, pick up knitting or other handwork that you can't do while smoking. Some people who like the feel of a cigarette in their mouths will suck on empty cigarette holders or pencils instead.

Count on success. At the outset, assume that this time you are going to succeed. But don't be consumed with guilt or feelings of failure if you backslide and take a cigarette. Chances of success improve each time you quit, so if you do backslide, simply start again with renewed determination and make an increased effort to avoid the previous pitfalls.

Rights of Nonsmokers

As noted earlier, tobacco smoke can be a major problem even for asthmatics who do not smoke. Fortunately, society is becoming more aware of the potential hazards of passive smoking and is increasingly sympathetic to the rights of non-smokers. Until recently, nonsmokers have truly been a silent majority. Although it may seem that "everyone smokes," the fact is three-fourths of all Americans do not smoke.

It is important to remember that efforts to protect the rights of nonsmokers are not a personal attack on smokers. Concern over the right to smoke-free air is no different from concern over any form of air pollution, and both smokers and nonsmokers endorse efforts to minimize pollution from to-bacco smoke. According to the American Lung Association, 78 percent of all people responding to a public opinion poll felt that employers had a right to ban all smoking on their premises. Surveys also have found that about 80 percent of nonsmokers would like to see smoking barred in more public places, and that just over half of smokers agree. Ninety per-cent of nonsmokers maintain that smoking is enough of a health hazard to warrant governmental action against it—a stand that 71 percent of smokers endorse.

Even so, many people with asthma and other conditions aggravated by tobacco smoke encounter problems from pas-sive smoking. The National Jewish patient handbook sug-gests the following steps that nonsmokers can take to counter the problem.

At work: In a polite but firm manner, let coworkers know that you object to their smoking. Suggest a survey of prefer-ences on no-smoking areas at work. Remember, a right to a no-smoking work area is now a legal concept.

At meetings: Propose no-smoking resolutions for clubs or organizations. Check into legal restrictions on smoking. In Colorado, for example, it is illegal to smoke in meeting rooms or waiting areas in state or local government-owned buildings. Where such laws exist, remind meeting planners or building managers of their provisions.

In restaurants: Request seating in a no-smoking area, even if there is none. Write a note on the bill requesting a non-smoking area. Such suggestions make management aware that there is a demand for a no-smoking section. Politely inform neighboring diners that their smoke is bothering you, or use body language—wave away smoke, grimace, move as far away as you can, and so on—to get your objection across.

Travel: Speak up when anyone violates no-smoking regulations on trains, planes, buses, elevators, and the like. Airlines can be fined $1,000 for noncompliance with a request for a no-smoking seat. Several major hotels have banned smoking entirely or have set aside no-smoking floors. When making reservations, ask about a hotel's smoking policies, and request accommodations in which guest smoking is not permitted.

At home: Ask people not to smoke in your home or designate a place, such as an outdoor porch or balcony, where those who must smoke can go. Write "Thank you for not smoking" on invitations and post a similar sign near the door where guests can see it.

Miscellaneous: Join no-smoking action groups (see list in Table 11). Support no-smoking legislation, and inform elected officials of the issues and your concern.

Table 11

Resources for Smoking Information and Programs

National Groups

American Lung Association
1740 Broadway
New York, N.Y. 10019
(212) 245-8000

Check white pages for local affiliates.

American Cancer Society
90 Park Avenue
New York, N.Y. 10016
(212) 736-3030

Check white pages for local affiliates.

American Heart Association
7320 Greenville Avenue
Dallas, Tex. 75231
(214) 750-5300

Check white pages for local affiliates.

Action on Smoking and Health (ASH)
2013 H Street, N.W.
Washington, D. C. 20006
(202) 659-4310

Public action group working for nonsmokers' rights.

Environmental Improvement Associates
109 Chestnut Street
Salem, N.J. 08079
(609) 935-4200

Organization working to eliminate tobacco smoke in workplace.

Nonsmokers Travel Club
8928 Bradmoor Drive
Bethesda, Md. 20034
(301) 530-1664

Organizes smoke-free tours in United States and abroad.

Smoke Signal
P.O. Box 99688
San Francisco, Calif. 94109
(415) 776-3739
Newsletter for nonsmokers.

To find local or state organizations, contact American Lung Association, American Cancer Society, or American Heart Association. Many states and cities have chapters of GASP (Groups Against Smoking Pollution), an organization devoted to enacting and enforcing laws protecting nonsmokers' rights.

CHAPTER 10
Exercise and Asthma

Many, if not most, people with asthma experience wheezing and other symptoms during exercise, especially if the exercise is of long duration and being done in the cold or windy outdoors. Frequently, asthmatic patients will not even be aware that exercise is a triggering factor, often because they simply lead sedentary lives. The young National Jewish patient who wanted to work on his stamp collection instead of joining others on a long walk is a typical example. The youth denied that asthma limited his activities, but questioning revealed that all his favorite pastimes were sedentary. When he was alone, he preferred to read or to work on his collections; with his friends, most time was spent playing computer games or just sitting around talking.

All of us experience feeling some shortness of breath when exercising at the peak of our endurance. This comes on quickly in someone who is in poor physical condition, or who has a heart or lung disorder that lowers the amount of oxygen available to body cells. In contrast, a person who is physically fit can exercise much longer—for example, run a marathon or jog for miles—without experiencing anything but normal tiredness. Asthmatics, including those who are in good physical shape, often find they start wheezing and feel very short of breath after a few minutes of exercise. Typically, a person with this problem will be able to exercise for six or seven minutes without difficulty, and then suddenly experience trouble in breathing. These symptoms are related more to asthmatic bronchospasm than to level of activity. The problem is likely to be worse when exercising under conditions that in themselves provoke asthma. For example, very cold air causes a degree of bronchospasm in even normal lungs—this is the body's way of protecting itself from undue exposure. Many asthmatics also are hypersensitive to wind, or very dry or very humid air (see Chapter 12).

Importance of Exercise Conditioning

People with asthma tend to be in poor physical condition for several reasons. Because vigorous physical activity is a common asthma trigger, many of them restrict their exercise to avoid the onset of symptoms. This sedentary life-style leads to a vicious cycle: The more sedentary a person, the poorer his or her physical condition, and the less tolerant to exercise he or she becomes. A person with poorly conditioned muscles and cardiovascular system does not use oxygen as efficiently as a person who is physically fit. Any increased workload makes the heart and lungs work harder. But if the person is experiencing exercise-induced bronchospasm, the lungs will not be able to meet the extra demand, resulting in earlier onset of shortness of breath. In addition to the lack of stamina, low cardiovascular reserve, and muscle weakness promoted by a sedentary life-style, asthma patients face an added risk. Many who have severe forms of the disease are on steroid medications, which, among other side effects, cause thinning of skin, muscle weakness, and *osteoporosis,* a thinning of the bones. Exercise promotes proper bone metabolism and helps keep bones strong. People with bone thinning, however, must exercise with caution to make sure that they do not put too much stress on weakened bones, since they are particularly vulnerable to stress fractures.

At National Jewish, exercise conditioning is an important part of the overall treatment program. "The trick is to break this sedentary cycle and to gradually build up the patient's exercise tolerance," Dr. Strunk explains.

As part of the initial work-up, most patients undergo exercise tolerance testing to measure both heart and pulmonary function. The patient is attached to an electrocardiogram machine, and then instructed to either walk on a treadmill or pedal a stationary exercise bicycle. The objective is to exercise until the heart rate reaches a certain number of beats per minute, and then to continue exercising for a specified period of time. (The test may be stopped if symptoms affecting either breathing or the heart's function occur.) During the test, an ear oximeter also may be attached to measure the amount of oxygen in the blood. Spirometry is done before starting, and then five to ten minutes after stopping. If there is no change in lung function, spirometry may be repeated twenty minutes after stopping the exercise. A drop in oxygen saturation of the blood, or a 20 percent reduction in FEV_1, are good indications of exercise-induced bronchospasm. It should be noted, however, that other lung disorders, such as emphysema, also may cause lowered blood oxygen during exercise.

To obtain as accurate test results as possible, patients are instructed not to take asthma medications beforehand. Specifically, patients should not use inhaled Intal (cromolyn) for two days; oral Alupent, Brethine, Proventil, or Ventolin for six hours: or inhaled Alupent, atropine, Brethine, Bronkosol, Proventil, or Ventolin for four hours. If the initial exercise challenge test indicates that physical activity is an asthma trigger, the test will be repeated at a later date; but this time, an inhaled anti-asthma medication will be given beforehand to determine whether this will prevent the bronchospasm.

Exercise Conditioning

Even among asthmatics whose wheezing is provoked by physical activity, exercise conditioning is a vital component of the overall treatment program at National Jewish. "Virtually every patient can benefit from exercise conditioning," says Dr. Strunk, himself an asthmatic who enjoys running, mountain climbing, and other vigorous activities. "Exercise not only improves cardiopulmonary fitness and increases stamina, it also provides important psychological benefits."

Cardiopulmonary fitness refers to the ability of the heart, lungs, and circulatory system to adapt during exercise so that the body's uptake of oxygen and output of carbon dioxide keep up with the muscles' consumption of oxygen and production of carbon dioxide. During vigorous aerobic exercise, the body's large muscles require increased oxygen and give off more carbon dioxide; if the heart and lungs cannot keep up with the demand, fatigue and shortness of breath result.

"Many of our patients, especially children, simply assume that they cannot participate in active games and are reluctant to even try," Dr. Strunk explains. "They come to us in woefully poor physical shape, not so much because of the limitations of their asthma as by their sedentary life-style and poor cardiopulmonary condition."

Still, most asthmatics, including children with severe forms of the disease, can increase their exercise tolerance by gradual exercise conditioning. This was demonstrated in a study of sixty-five young National Jewish patients. At the outset, forty of the sixty-five were unable to exercise at a rate considered normal for their age, sex, and size. To determine their fitness level, the children, who were eight to seventeen years old, were tested on bicycle ergometers. The goal was to achieve 85 percent of the maximal heart rate for the youngster's age, size, and sex; children who could exercise at this level were considered physically fit and encouraged to participate in swimming, active games, and/or sports. Those who could not exercise at 85 percent of their predicted capacity were referred for physical conditioning.

Exercise conditioning consisted of working out on the bicycle ergometers for twelve minutes a day, five days a week. An exercise goal was set for each session, such as, for example, reaching a heart rate of 120 beats per minute. A physical therapist would measure the patient's heart rate before each session. To prevent asthma symptoms, the patients would use a bronchodilator medication before the sessions. The physical therapist would gradually increase the ergometer workload until the patient reached 60 to 75 percent of the normal maximal heart rate. As a rule of thumb, the maximal heart rate is determined by subtracting age from 220; thus the average maximal heart rate for a 16-year-old would be 204 beats per minute. The conditioning target zone is usually 70 to 85 percent of this; in this example, 142 to 173 beats per minute. However, a lower conditioning zone of 60 to 80 percent may be used for patients with heart or lung disorders. (Table 12 shows how to calculate maximal and conditioning heart rates.) In the beginning, a patient may be able to exercise only for five or six minutes at 60 or 65 percent of the maximal rate. In a National Jewish exercise study of children with asthma, some were very severely restricted and could exercise at less than 30 percent of their predicted heart rate. Others were in good shape, and could exercise well above their predicted rate. By the time they left the hospital, 84 percent of those who had been below the norm in the beginning were able to achieve normal exercise ranges; only two of the patients failed to show improvement in their fitness levels, insisting that they were too fatigued during the exercise sessions to continue.

Table 12
How to Determine Your Heart's Target Zone
Formula: 220 minus your age, multiplied by 60 to 80 percent

AGE	AVERAGE MAXIMUM HEART RATE	TARGET ZONE 60%	80%
15	205	123	164
20	200	120	160
25	195	117	156
30	190	114	152
35	185	111	148
40	180	108	144
45	175	105	140
50	170	102	136
55	165	99	132
60	160	96	128
65	155	93	124
70	150	90	120

At the conclusion of the study, the National Jewish researchers wrote: "This study demonstrates that a high proportion of children with severe asthma have abnormal cardiopulmonary fitness levels. . . . Nearly all of the patients made significant gains in cardiopulmonary fitness after the bicycle ergometry conditioning program. . . . The magnitude of the gains was not related to improvements in pulmonary function achieved during the training periods. . . . [Instead,] the most important variable in determining success was length of training (three to five times a week for three to six weeks) and not other underlying abnormalities." In short, the youngsters who stayed with their conditioning training, no matter how difficult it was, were rewarded with marked improvement in stamina and endurance. Although most of the youngsters did well in group sessions, there were some that needed individual encouragement to push themselves. The fact that the conditioning took place in a closely supervised hospital setting in which it was taken for granted that all of the children would participate also undoubtedly contributed to the marked improvement. Even so, the lesson for all children with asthma is clear: Inactivity breeds further inactivity and disability. The ability to achieve improved physical condition is unrelated to the severity of the asthma, which usually can be controlled during exercise by preventive inhaled medication and, if needed, supplemental oxygen.

Conditioning in Adults

Of course, adults with asthma can benefit from exercise conditioning just as much as children can. Not uncommonly, the problems resulting from inactivity are even greater in adults than in children—they have had more years for the sedentary life-style to take its toll, and long-term use of steroids may have contributed further to bone thinning and muscle weakness. Repeatedly, doctors at National Jewish stress that there is no truth to the statement: "Because you have a lung problem, you should take it easy." In fact, just the opposite is true.

The National Jewish fitness conditioning program for adults is similar to that for children, but many adult patients also require special exercises to increase muscle tone and strength. Individualized programs are developed according to specific problems. To strengthen leg muscles, for example, leg lifts using ankle weights may be recommended. Stretching exercises may be needed to improve flexibility. Bicycle ergometers are used to improve cardiopulmonary conditioning.

Picking the Right Exercises

Although most patients begin to notice a marked improvement within weeks, regular vigorous exercise must be continued to maintain the gains. And this is where most would-be exercisers, including people with no pulmonary or other health problems, regress. After a few weeks or months, they begin to backslide, cutting back on their exercise sessions until they once again lapse into their former sedentary ways. To maintain physical fitness, it is absolutely necessary to exercise at 60 to 80 percent of the maximum heart rate for fifteen to thirty minutes at least three (and preferably five) times a week.

In general, people with asthma can participate in most types of physical activity, although some may encounter problems with high-endurance activities such as running a marathon. Swimming seems to be one of the best activities for asthmatic patients. The humid environment helps prevent bronchoconstriction, the water eases stress on weight-bearing joints, and the swimming can be paced to provide the right combination of aerobic exercise and resting while almost every muscle in the body is being worked. Brisk walking is another ideal exercise; in some respects, it may be better than swimming because it can be done by almost everyone without requiring any skills or any equipment other than a comfortable pair of shoes. A walking program can be tailored to meet individual needs and limitations, including those of people with severe asthma, emphysema, and bronchitis.

The National Jewish patient handbook recommends brisk, aerobic walking—defined as walking at a pace vigorous enough to increase the heart rate to 60 to 80 percent of its maximum—for fifteen to thirty minutes three to seven times a week. "It should become a routine, year-round, lifelong activity," the handbook urges. Almost everyone can find an appropriate place to walk—around the neighborhood, at a shopping mall, along a country road or seaside beach, at a local high school track, "Y," or health club. Each individual has his or her favorite time of day for walking: Some find that an early morning walk is an ideal way to wake up and get the day off to a brisk start; others prefer walking at midday to prevent overeating at lunch and to gain a renewed burst of energy for the afternoon; still others like to unwind with a long evening walk. Taking a walk can ease feelings of "the blues," or counter the effects of stress. Walking is also a good way to help control weight—regular exercise both burns up calories and also helps keep the appetite in check.

When engaging in aerobic walking or other exercise, you should remember the following:

- Wear comfortable walking or running shoes.

- Take a pre-exercise medication, if one has been prescribed.

- Stretch before you set out, and do cool-down stretching exercises at the end of the exercise session.

- Start slowly and pace yourself, especially in the beginning.

- Breathe deeply and evenly.

- Take your pulse before beginning; again after walking about ten minutes (or if you feel tired); and, finally, after exercising. The heart rate should be within the target zone of 60 to 80 percent of your maximum heart rate (see Table 12); if it is too slow, speed up, and if it is too fast, slow down. Try to walk for twelve to twenty minutes with your heart rate in the target zone.

- Stop if you experience dizziness, wheezing, shortness of breath, a racing heartbeat, chest pains, nausea, faint or light-headed feelings, or other symptoms. Consult your doctor, especially if the symptoms persist.

People who experience symptoms during adverse weather conditions—for example, when it is cold, or damp and rainy, or hot and humid, or during periods of air pollution, high pollen, and so on—would do better to exercise indoors. Under these conditions, pedaling an exercise bicycle or ergometer, and using a rowing machine or other equipment, may be preferable to exercising outdoors. Also, most people can find an appropriate place to walk indoors.

Before undertaking an exercise program, it is a good idea to consult your doctor first. Although virtually everyone can benefit from exercise conditioning, people with heart disease and those with certain types of lung disorders may need to use certain precautions and select their pace and type of activity with care.

Be patient. You have had a sedentary lifetime in which to get out of shape; it is unrealistic to expect to see results overnight. Even so, most people notice a marked improvement after only a week or two on an exercise program. They find it easier to climb a flight of stairs and they have more energy at the end of the day. The psychological benefits of exercise conditioning also are well known. People who have begun to engage in consistent exercise report that they enjoy an enhanced sense of well-being; that they are not as irritable or easily depressed as they were previously. These benefits can be particularly important for asthmatics or other victims of a chronic disease; they promote a greater sense of control and mastery over one's life. And all at no cost except a little shoe leather and a half-hour a day that might otherwise have been spent staring at TV!

CHAPTER 11

Foods and Asthma

For some asthmatics, especially children, there is a clear relationship between asthma and certain foods. But tracking down the specific foods and eliminating them from the diet often require patience and considerable detective work. If the reaction is immediate—for example, if a child invariably starts to cough or wheeze after eating a particular food—the matter can be fairly straightforward. Confirm the sensitivity to the substance by a diagnostic test and then eliminate it from his or her diet. Unfortunately, it is not always this simple; the reaction may not be immediate, with symptoms appearing an hour or two after a meal. In addition, the problem may not be from the food itself, but from additives or contaminants in it, such as molds, antibiotic residues, dyes, flavoring, or preservatives.

What Is a Food Allergy?

Many people confuse food allergies with food intolerance, toxicity, and other very different reactions. The confusion is compounded by the fact that even doctors do not always use the same term to describe a particular response.

The accompanying table of definitions was recently published by the American Academy of Allergy and Immunology's Committee on Adverse Reactions to Foods. From this table you will see that a food allergy, a term synonymous with *food hypersensitivity,* entails an immune-system response, in which antibodies are produced against a specific food antigen.

Table 13

Definitions of Terms Used in Describing Adverse Reactions to Foods

TERM	DEFINITION
Adverse food reaction	A clinically abnormal response believed due to a food or food additive
Food sensitivity	A general term implying an adverse reaction to a food or food additive
Food hypersensitivity	An immunologic hypersensitivity or truly allergic reaction resulting from consuming a food or food additive
Food allergy	A term synonymous with food hypersensitivity, but frequently overused and applied to an adverse reaction
Anaphylactoid reaction to a food	Anaphylaxis-like food reaction as a result of a nonimmune release of chemical mediators that can mimic a food hypersensitivity
Food idiosyncrasy	An abnormal response to a food or food additive which may be similar to a hypersensitivity reaction but does not involve the immune system
Food toxicity	A general term implying an adverse reaction following ingestion of a food or food additive as a result of a direct nonimmune response
Food poisoning	An adverse reaction following food ingestion that is a result of a natural toxic constituent of

TERM	DEFINITION
	food, or contamination of the food by micro-organisms and/or their toxins
Pharmacologic food reaction	A reaction as a result of a chemical in food or food additives
Metabolic food reaction	A metabolic response to food or food additives

(Adapted from *American Academy of Allergy and Immunology Committee on Adverse Reactions to Foods,* National Institute of Allergy and Infectious Diseases, U.S. Dept. of Health & Human Services, 1984.)

As discussed in earlier chapters, classic IgE-mediated allergic responses involve *mast cells,* which are particularly abundant in the gastrointestinal tract, the lungs, and the skin; and *basophils,* which circulate in the blood. Because of the high concentrations of mast cells in the intestines, lungs, and skin, it logically follows that these organs are the most likely to experience symptoms of an immediate allergic reaction. Thus, a food allergy may cause swelling, tingling, and burning in the mouth and nasal passages, nausea, vomiting, intestinal cramps, gas, diarrhea, and other such symptoms; skin itching, rashes, swelling and hives, runny nose, and the swelling of the larynx or bronchospasms characteristic of asthma. These symptoms, which often take place immediately or within two hours of eating, may occur in a wide variety of combinations and widely varying degrees of severity, ranging from the barely noticeable all the way to a life-threatening anaphylaxis.

Frequently, the asthmatic with food allergies will have other allergic symptoms. For example, a child may have chronic sinusitis, which in itself can provoke asthma. Many asthmatic children also suffer from chronic middle ear problems. Eczema or frequent bouts of diarrhea and other intestinal upsets are still other tip-offs that the problem may be related to allergies.

Diagnosis

Often the source of a food allergy can be detected simply by questioning and observing. For example, a child may make an association that the parents overlook. Refusal to eat a particular food because "it makes my mouth burn" or "it makes me sick" should not be ignored; it could be that the youngster has figured out the source of his or her problem and is trying to eliminate it from the diet. Keeping a food and symptom diary also may be helpful; if coughing, wheezing, and other symptoms invariably occur on days that a child has had eggs or nuts, for example, this may well indicate that these foods contain allergens that are provoking his or her asthma.

A number of tests may be used to confirm a food allergy, with varying degrees of success or relevancy. Skin tests, when properly done and interpreted, can demonstrate an IgE-mediated sensitivity to foods. The method favored by National Jewish doctors entails placing a drop of food extract on the skin, using a needle to lightly puncture the skin, and allowing a small amount of the extract to penetrate it. If a wheal—a reddened bump in the skin—of three millimeters or more in diameter appears in fifteen minutes, the test is considered positive. Care must be taken not to introduce too much extract into the skin because this can cause an irritation that may be misinterpreted as a true allergic reaction. It also should be noted that a positive skin test does not necessarily mean that the person will experience clinical symptoms; some people will test positive to a variety of foods, yet not have any symptoms when eating them. However, the absence of a positive skin test for a suspected food makes the diagnosis of an IgE-mediated sensitivity to that food extremely unlikely.

A RAST test, a laboratory procedure to measure levels of IgE antibodies against specific antigens in a person's serum, is not as sensitive as a skin test, and is also more expensive. Still, it may be recommended for patients in whom skin testing is not advisable; for example, a person with widespread skin disorders or the rare individual who is so sensitive to a substance that a skin test might be hazardous.

Elimination diets, in which suspected foods are removed from the diet and the person is expected to watch for any subsequent improvement in symptoms, also may be useful in determining whether a suspected food is producing symptoms. A child with a suspected milk allergy, for example, would have all milk and milk products removed from his or her diet. The child would then be carefully observed for one or two weeks to see if the symptoms lessened. If there is an improvement, it still does not necessarily mean that milk was causing the problem. To verify this, milk will be reintroduced into the diet to see if the symptoms recur. This approach is recommended if there is no great urgency to identify the offending substances, and works best if only one or two foods are suspected allergens. Otherwise, the elimination diet may be overly and unnecessarily restrictive to the point where it interferes with good nutrition. Dr. Dan Atkins, a National Jewish allergist, recalled a thirteen-year-old patient whose mother was convinced that her son was allergic to a large number of foods. Eventually, the youngster's diet was so restricted that he was allowed only seven or eight foods. His asthma persisted, and in addition to his pulmonary problems, the boy was seriously malnourished when he arrived at National Jewish.

"Our testing failed to confirm that this child was allergic to any of the foods on the mother's list, even though both mother and son were convinced that he could not tolerate most of the components needed for a healthful diet," Dr. Atkins recalled. Although elimination diets can sometimes be tried by patients on their own, it is a good idea to seek the guidance of a board-certified allergist. Seemingly different foods are often chemically related, and as noted earlier, the problem may not be in the food itself, but in a dye or other additive. In addition, a number of studies have shown that the suspected relationship between the ingestion of a certain food and the development of symptoms could not be proven by thorough investigation. Thus, foods are often mistakenly incriminated as the cause of symptoms.

Blind food challenges are the most reliable tests to verify whether a particular food or foods are responsible for an allergic reaction. This test entails provoking a reaction by giving the patient a suspected food and then observing for symptoms. This may be done openly, in which case both the patient and the observer know which foods are being tested; or blindly, in which case neither is aware of the food. In a double-blind challenge, the suspected food may be given at one time and a placebo at another and the responses are then compared.

Blind or double-blind challenges are likely to produce the most accurate results because neither the patient nor the observer can bias the results. For example, the thirteen-year-old patient described by Dr. Atkins was certain he could not tolerate dozens of different foods. When he was openly given these foods, he would start coughing and experiencing other symptoms. But when freeze-dried samples of these same foods were given in capsules during blind and double-blind challenges, he experienced none of these symptoms. Nor did skin tests reveal any sensitivity. In such a case, the conclusion is obvious: something other than the suspected food or foods is provoking the asthma. In contrast, the production of symptoms after eating the offending food, but not the placebo, confirms that the person is indeed allergic to that particular food.

As with all allergy tests, food challenges must be conducted with care and precision to avoid getting biased results or, in the case of hypersensitivity, provoking a medical emergency. The food or food extracts must be given in adequate amounts; administering several pills of dried foods may be necessary to provide enough of the offending substance to provoke symptoms. In rare instances, dehydration may alter the allergen in such a way that the body will not react to it; thus, blinded food challenges with freeze-dried foods in capsules should always be followed by an open challenge with a regular portion of the suspected food in its natural state. Obviously, challenge tests should be done under careful medical supervision.

A number of other diagnostic tests have been proposed to detect food allergies. These include the use of sublingual food drops, in which extracts of the suspected allergen are placed on the tongue and the person is observed for symptoms; cytotoxic food testing, in which food extracts are added to white cells extracted from fresh blood drawn from the patient and the cells observed for changes; and titration neutralization skin testing, in which varying doses of a suspected allergen are injected into the skin to find a dose that will "neutralize" a patient's symptoms. None of these methods have been scientifically proven, and although they are widely touted in the popular media as being safe and reliable, they are not recommended by the American Academy of Allergy and Immunology.

Common Food Allergens

Obviously, almost any food or family of foods may provoke an allergic response in persons who have developed sufficient antibodies against them. But some foods are known to be more allergenic than others. These include eggs (particularly egg whites), cow's milk, shellfish and other seafoods, nuts, wheat, and corn. An allergy to one member of a food family may mean a person is allergic to other members of the same family. Table 14 lists food families and their principal foods.

Table 14
Families of Foods

ANIMAL GROUPS

1. Amphibians
   - frog

2. Birds (flesh and organs)
   - chicken
   - Cornish hen
   - duck
   - goose
   - grouse
   - guinea hen (fowl)
   - partridge
   - pheasant
   - pigeon
   - quail
   - squab
   - turkey

3. Crustaceans
   - crab
   - crayfish
   - lobster
   - prawn
   - shrimp

4. Eggs (bird)
   - ovomucoid
   - ovovitellin
   - white
   - whole
   - yolk

5. Fish (representative families)
   - Acipenseridae
     - sturgeon (caviar)
   - Anguillidae
     - eel
   - Argentinidae
     - smelt
   - Carangidae
     - pompano
   - Centrarchidae
     - black bass
     - crappie
     - sunfish
   - Clupeidae
     - herring
     - sardine
     - shad
     - sprat
   - Cyprinidae
     - carp

ANIMAL GROUPS

5. Fish (continued)
    Esocidae
      muscallonge
      pickerel
      pike
    Gadidae
      cod
      haddock
      hake
      pollack
      scrod
    Mugilidae
      mullet
    Percidae
      perch
    Pleuronectidae
      flounder
      halibut
    Salmonidae
      grayling
      salmon
      trout
      whitefish
    Scienidae
      croaker
      drum
      redfish
      sea trout
      weakfish
    Scombridae
      bonito
      mackerel
      tuna
    Serranidae
      grouper
      rockfish
      white bass
    Siluridae
      bullhead
      catfish
    Soleidae
      sole

5. Fish (continued)
    Sparidae
      porgy
      red snapper
    Stolephoridae
      anchovy
    Xyphidae
      swordfish

6. Red Meats (flesh and internal organs)
    a.   Bovidae
        Cow
          beef
          calf
          steer
          veal
        Gelatin
        Goat
        Ox
        Sheep
          lamb
          mutton
        Sweetbread
    b.   Suidae (pig)
          bacon
          boar
          ham
          hog
          pig
          pork
          sausage
          scrapple
          sow
          swine

7. Milk products (cow, goat)
        butter
        buttermilk
        casein
        cheese

ANIMAL GROUPS

7. Milk products (continued)
    cream
      sour
      whipped
    ice cream
    lactalbumin
    milk
      condensed
      evaporated
      homogenized
      powdered
      raw
      skimmed
    selected infant
    formulas
    yogurt

8. Mollusks
    abalone
    clam
    cockle
    mussel
    octopus
    oyster
    quahog
    scallop
    snail (escargot)
    squid

9. Reptiles
    alligator
    crocodile
    rattlesnake
    terrapin
    turtle

PLANT GROUPS

10. Apple family
    apple

10. Apple family (continued)
      cider
      vinegar (apple cider)
    crab apple
    pear
    quince
    quince seed

11. Banana family
    banana*
    plantain

12. Beech family
    beechnut
    chestnut
    chinquapin

13. Birch family
    filbert
    hazelnut
    wintergreen *(Betula spp.)*

14. Buckwheat family
    buckwheat
    rhubarb
    sorrel

15. Cashew family
    cashew
    mango
    pistachio

16. Citrus family
    citron
    grapefruit
    kumquat
    lemon
    lime
    orange

PLANT GROUPS

16. Citrus family (continued)
    tangelo
    tangerine

17. Cola nut family

    chocolate (cocoa)
    cola (kola) nut

18. Fungi

    mushroom
    truffle
    yeast
      baker's
      brewer's
      distiller's
      Fleischmann's
      lactose-fermenting
      lager beer

19. Ginger family

    cardamom (cardamon,
      cardamum)
    East Indian arrowroot
    ginger
    turmeric

20. Goosefoot family

    beet
    lamb's quarters
    spinach
    Swiss chard

21. Gourd (melon) family

    cantaloupe
      (muskmelon)*
    casaba (winter
      muskmelon)
    Chinese watermelon
    citron melon
    cucumber

21. Gourd family (continued)
    gherkin
    honeydew melon
    Persian melon
    pumpkin
    summer squash
    watermelon*
    winter squash

22. Grape family

    champagne
    grape
    raisin
    vinegar (wine)
    wine (grape)

23. Grass (cereal) family

    bamboo
    barley
    corn (maize)
    hominy
    malt (germinated
      grain)
    millet
    oat
    popcorn
    rice
    rye
    sorghum
    sugar cane
    wheat
      bran
      germ
      gliadin
      globulin
      glutenin
      leucosin
      proteose
      whole

PLANT GROUPS

24. Heath family
    black huckleberry
    blueberry
    cranberry
    wintergreen *(Pyrola spp.)*

25. Laurel family
    avocado
    bay leaf
    cinnamon
    sassafras

26. Lecythis family
    Brazil nut

27. Lily family
    aloe
    asparagus
    chives
    garlic
    leek
    onion
    sarsaparilla
    shallot

28. Madder family
    coffee

29. Mallow family
    cottonseed
    marshmallow
    okra (gumbo)

30. Mint family
    balm
    basil
    catnip
    horehound

30. Mint family (continued)
    Japanese artichoke
    lavender
    marjoram
    mint
    oregano
    peppermint
    rosemary
    sage
    savory
    spearmint
    thyme

31. Morning glory family
    sweet potato
    yam

32. Mulberry family
    breadfruit
    breadnut
    fig
    hop

33. Mustard family
    broccoli
    Brussels sprouts
    cabbage
    cauliflower
    collards
    garden cress
    horseradish
    kale
    kohlrabi
    mustard
    radish
    rutabaga
    turnip
    watercress

PLANT GROUPS

34. Myrtle family
    allspice
    clove
    guava
    myrtle
    pimento

35. Nightshade family
    bell pepper
    cayenne pepper
    chili (paprika) (red pepper)
    eggplant
    ground cherry
    melon pear
    potato (white)
    strawberry tomato
    tobacco
    tomato
    tree tomato

36. Nutmeg family
    mace
    nutmeg

37. Olive family
    jasmine
    olive

38. Orchid family
    vanilla

39. Palm family
    cabbage palm
    coconut
    date

40. Papaya family
    papain
    papaya

41. Parsley family
    anise
    caraway
    carrot
    celeriac
    celery
    coriander
    dill
    fennel
    parsley
    parsnip

42. Pea (legume) family
    acacia
    alfalfa
    black-eyed pea (cowpea)
    broad bean (fava bean)
    carob bean (St. John's bread)
    chick pea (garbanzo)
    common bean
        kidney
        navy
        pinto
        string (green)
    Jack bean
    lentil
    licorice
    lima bean
    mesquite
    pea
    peanut

PLANT GROUPS

42. Pea family (continued)
   soybean
   tamarind
   tragacanth

43. Pepper family
   black pepper

44. Pine family
   juniper
   pine nut (Pignolia)

45. Pineapple family
   pineapple

46. Plum family
   almond
   apricot
   cherry
   peach, nectarine
   plum, prune

47. Poppy family
   poppyseed

48. Rose family
   black raspberry
   blackberry
   boysenberry,
   dewberry, loganberry
   red raspberry

Rose family (continued)
   strawberry

49. Saxifrage family
   currant, gooseberry

50. Sunflower family
   (composite**, aster)
   absinthe (sagebrush,
   wormwood)
   artichoke
   camomile
   chicory
   dandelion
   endive, escarole
   Jerusalem artichoke
   lettuce
   oyster plant (salsify)
   safflower
   sunflower seed
   tansy
   tarragon

51. Tea family

52. Walnut family
   black walnut
   butternut
   English walnut
   hickory nut
   pecan

---

* Reported palatal itching and swelling in ragweed-sensitive patients after ingestion of melons and bananas has no basis in similarity of food groups, nor do these fruits have antigens that cross-react with ragweed antigen E.

** Members of the family Compositae have cross-reacting antigens with members of the family Ambrosiaceae, of which ragweed is a member. This shared property explains reactions, for example, to ingestion of camomile tea in ragweed-sensitive individuals. (Similarly, ragweed-sensitive patients may react to pyrethrum, an insecticide made from chrysanthemums, members of the family Compositae. This reaction is not food-related, however.)

(From *Adverse Reactions to Foods*, American Academy of Allergy and Immunology Committee on Adverse Reactions to Foods and the National Insitute of Allergy and Infectious Diseases, U.S. Dept. of Health and Human Services, NIH Publication 84-2442, 1984.)

Just as important as the basic foods are substances that may be added to them in processing or cooking, such as preservatives. Some people react to salicylates, which are present in many foods. See Table 15 for sources of salicylates.)

Table 15

Sources of Salicylates

FOOD

Beverages:	Tea, root beer, birch beer
Meat:	Corned beef, meat processed with vinegar
Fat:	Salad dressing, mayonnaise, avocado, olives
Starch:	White potatoes, products with potato starch
Vegetables:	Cucumbers, green pepper and other peppers, tomatoes
Fruits:	Apples, apple cider, apricots, blackberries, boysenberries, cherries, currants, dewberries, gooseberries, huckleberries, maraschino cherries, grapes, melon, nectarines, peaches, raisins, raspberries, prunes, plums
Sweets/Desserts:	Any mint or wintergreen product
Miscellaneous:	Cloves, pickles, catsup, tartar sauce, Tabasco sauce, cider vinegar, beer, wine, distilled alcoholic beverages (except vodka), or any product containing any restricted food item

DRUGS

Acetidine	Bufferin	Liquiprin
Alka-Seltzer	Coricidin	Midol
Anacin	Darvon Compound	Pepto-Bismol
Anahist	Dristan	Persistin
A.C.P.	Ecotrin	Sal-Sayne
Aspirin	Empirin Compound	Stanback
BC	Excedrin	Theracin
Bromo-Quinine	4-Way Cold Capsules	Trigesic
Bromo-Seltzer	Inhiston	

FLAVORING

Antiseptics	Cosmetics	Oil of Wintergreen
Beverages	Gum	Perfumes
Breath Sweeteners	Lozenges	Toothpaste
Candies	Mouthwash	

PLANTS

Aspens	Acacia	Camellia
Birches	Spirea	Hyacinth
Poplars	Teaberry	Marigold
Willows	Calycanthus	Milkwort

SUNTAN LOTIONS AND OILS

Acetyl Salicylic Acid	Procaine Salicylate
Aluminum Acetyl Salicylate	Sal Ethyl Carbonate
Ammonium Salicylate	Salicylamide
Arthropan	Salicylsalicylic Acid
Calcium Acetyl Salicylate	Santy (Santalyl Salicylate)
Choline Salicylate	Sodium Salicylate
Ethyl Salicylate	Stronclate
Lithium Salicylate	Strontium Salicylate
Methyl Salicylate	
Para Amino Salicylate	
Phenyl Salicylate	

MISCELLANEOUS

Methylene Desalicylic Acid (used in lubricating oils)
Salicylanilide (anti-mildew)

Soap (with green or wintergreen fragrance)
Sulfosalicyclic Acid (chemical)

(From *Pride, Reference Manual for the Nurse Educator,* National Jewish
Center for Immunology and Respiratory Medicine, Denver, Colo., 1985.)

Most people are familiar with the "Chinese restaurant
syndrome," a constellation of headaches and other symptoms
related to the MSG (monosodium glutamate) that is used
liberally in Chinese and many other cuisines. Sulfitic agents,
which are used as antioxidants to prevent browning or other
discoloration and to inhibit the growth of certain microorganisms during fermentation, also are common allergens.
Sulfites pose a particularly serious threat to asthmatics since
they have been linked to a number of deaths from anaphylactic reactions. The Food and Drug Administration has ruled
that foods containing sulfites must be labeled as such, but this
does not remove the risk people encounter when eating in
restaurants, salad bars, and other places where the chemicals
are commonly used. Also, many wines and fermented foods
contain sulfites, and may not be labeled as such. Tables 16
and 17 were prepared by staff members at National Jewish;
Table 16 lists foods that commonly contain sulfites, and Table
17 outlines a model sulfite-free diet.

Table 16

Foods Containing Sulfitic Agents

The following is a list of foods which contain sulfitic agent(s). The list is not all-inclusive and the ingredients should be verified for contents on all food items.

BREADS/CRACKERS

Pillsbury Quick Bread Mix:

> Carrot Nut—dried carrots (color protected with sodium sulfite and sodium bisulfite)

> Apricot Nut—dried apricot pieces (color protected with sulfur dioxide)

> Nabisco Swiss Cheese Crackers—sodium sulfite added

CAKES

Betty Crocker Snackin' Cake Mix:

> Applesauce Raisin—sodium bisulfite

> Carrot Nut—dried carrots (color protected with sodium sulfite and sodium bisulfite)

Betty Crocker Super Moist Cake Mix:

> Apple Cinnamon—dried apples (sodium bisulfite)

> Carrot Cake—dried carrots (sodium sulfite)

Pillsbury Apple 'n Streusel Coffee Cake—dried apples (sodium bisulfite)

Pillsbury Apple Turnover—dried apples (sodium bisulfite)

Pillsbury Plus Cake Mix:

> Carrot 'n Spice—dried carrots (color protected with sodium sulfite)

MEAT OR MEAT SUBSTITUTE

Betty Crocker Hamburger Helper

> (color and freshness preserved by sodium sulfite):

Cheeseburger Macaroni, Chili Tomato, Hamburger Potato Au Gratin, Lasagna and Tamale Pie Flavors

Betty Crocker Tuna Helper (color and freshness preserved by sodium sulfite)

POTATO OR POTATO SUBSTITUTE

Betty Crocker Potato Mix—dried potatoes (color preserved by sodium bisulfite):

Au Gratin, Creamed, Hashed Browns, Hickory Smoke Cheese, Julienne, Potato Buds, Scalloped and Sour Cream 'n Chive Flavors

Betty Crocker Noodles Almondine Mix (color and freshness preserved by sodium sulfite)

Pillsbury Hungry Jack Mashed Potato Mix—sodium bisulfite

Stove Top Stuffing Mix:

Chicken Flavor—dried celery (with sodium sulfite added as preservative)

Pork Flavor—dried celery (with sulfur dioxide added as preservative)

With Rice—dried celery (with sulfur dioxide added as preservative)

Uncle Ben's The Original Long Grain & Wild Rice—sodium sulfite, sodium bisulfite as preservative for vegetables

SALAD DRESSINGS

Good Seasons Salad Dressing Mix (sodium bisulfite added):

Cheese Italian, Italian, low Calorie Italian, Riviera French and Zesty Italian

Good Seasons Salad Dressing Mix (sulfur dioxide added):

Buttermilk Farm Style

French's Meatloaf Seasoning Mix—dried potatoes (sodium sulfite added to preserve quality)

Schilling Dehydrated Flakes (sulfite added):
   Celery, Sweet Pepper, and Vegetable

(From *Pride, Reference Manual for the Nurse Educator,* National Jewish Center for Immunology and Respiratory Medicine, Denver, Colo., 1985.)

Table 17
Sulfite-Free Diet

This diet is designed to minimize the intake of sulfitic agents. These agents include potassium metabisulfite, potassium bisulfite, sodium metabisulfite, sodium bisulfite, sodium sulfite, and sulfur dioxide. These sulfitic agents are used in the food-processing industry and function as: (1) preservatives to reduce or prevent microbial spoilage of foods; (2) antioxidants to minimize discoloration of foods; (3) inhibitors of undesirable microorganizisms during fermentation; and (4) sanitizing agents for fermentation equipment.

The highest consumption occurs when consuming restaurant salads sprayed with metabisulfite. Other main sources include dehydrated fruits and vegetables, wine, and beer. (*Most significant sources indicated below.)

FOOD GROUP	FOODS TO AVOID
Milk	None
Meat	*Shrimp and other shellfish, dried fish
Eggs	None
Cheese	None
Bread	Commercial bread mixes that contain dried fruits. Used as a dough conditioner in pizza and pie crust.
Cereal	Cereals that contain dried fruits
Potato or Substitute	*Dehydrated or instant potatoes. Rice or noodle mixes that contain dehydrated vegetables. Bread stuffing mixes.

FOOD GROUP	FOODS TO AVOID
Vegetables	*Dried vegetables and commercial products containing dried vegetables. In restaurants avoid vegetable mixes and salad bars that have been sprayed or dipped with metabisulfite. Vegetable juices, guacamole.
Fruits	*Light-colored dried fruits and commercial products containing dried fruits. In restaurants avoid fresh fruits that may have been sprayed or dipped in metabisulfite. Fresh California grapes.
Soup	Dehydrated or instant soup mixes.
Fats	None
Desserts/Sweets	Any commercial products containing ingredients not allowed.
Seasonings	Seasonings containing dehydrated vegetables. Olives, hot peppers.
Beverages	*Carbonated beverages with sulfur dioxide. Wine and beer. Fruit beverages such as grape soda.

(From *Pride, Reference Manual for the Nurse Educator,* National Jewish Center for Immunology and Respiratory Medicine, Denver, Colo., 1985.)

Contaminants in Foods

Foods may contain many contaminants that provoke adverse reactions. Examples include a variety of molds, antibiotics, pesticides, and insect parts. A person may be allergic to certain cheeses and yet not have problems with milk or other milk products. In such instances, the molds used to make the cheese may be the culprits. Table 18 lists common foods that contain molds. People who are sensitive to ragweed may react to residues of pryethrum, an insecticide made from chrysanthemums, a member of the same family as ragweed. The possibility of a contaminant should always be considered when a person suffers a reaction to a food he or she usually tolerates without problems.

Table 18

Foods That Commonly Contain Molds

- Cheeses of all kinds, sour cream, sour milk, and buttermilk
- Mushrooms
- Soy sauce and all products containing vinegar, including mayonnaise, catsup, pickles, etc.
- Alcoholic beverages, including wine and beer
- Pumpernickel bread and other sourdough breads and those made with large amounts of yeast
- Smoked or pickled meats and fish, including sausages and hot dogs
- Sauerkraut and other fermented or pickled foods
- Dried fruits, including raisins
- Any meat or other food that has been left standing for more than a day or so. Refrigeration retards but does not prevent the growth of molds.

Practical Pointers

Dealing with food allergies can be very frustrating, especially in those rare cases where a large number of foods are involved. A child who is allergic to milk products is going to feel deprived—and inclined to cheat—when his or her friends all are enjoying ice cream at a birthday party. Sometimes a small amount of the offending food can be tolerated. For example, if a child's allergy to milk is mild, he or she may be able to tolerate a piece of cake in which milk is an ingredient. But this should be determined beforehand by experimenting at home. Of course, such experiments should not be tried if the child has had severe reactions when exposed to the substance.

Many foods are not what they seem to be. For example, an allergy to walnuts eliminates not only the nuts but also foods in which walnut oil or flour may be used, without the person knowing it. Walnut oil may be used in salad dressings and other foods that are not ordinarily associated with nuts. Restaurant eating can pose special problems, because quite often a waiter has no idea of the ingredients that make up a particular dish. You often have to go directly to the chef or manager to find out if a particular food is, indeed, safe. Is this really important? Assuredly yes, especially if you or a family member has a serious hypersensitivity. Each year, a number of deaths occur from food reactions.

Reading food labels and interpreting a variety of terms becomes a mandatory exercise. A child with food allergies may be better off bringing a lunch from home rather than trying to cope with what is served at school. Even if the school lunch personnel are given a list of forbidden foods, mix-ups can occur. Similarly, whenever the child is eating away from home, the person preparing the food should be given very specific lists. Simply saying "Johnny cannot have milk" is not enough, because many people forget that milk products come in many forms and are in a wide range of foods.

Not uncommonly, an important source of nutrients, such as milk, must be eliminated from the diet. A dietitian or doctor experienced in nutrition can offer guidance on substitutes that will provide the missing nutrients. But if an entire group of foods cannot be tolerated, supplements may be needed to protect against deficiencies.

When facing the frustrations and challenges of eliminating favored foods from a child's diet, parents often despair that it simply will not be possible for the regimen to be adhered to. It may not be easy to do; after all, asthma and its treatment can be frustrating. But if following a particular diet makes breathing easier, this reward alone should provide sufficient motivation for the child to make the needed sacrifices.

CHAPTER 12
Weather and Asthma

Many of us have an aunt or other elderly relative who can predict a change in the weather because her arthritis is "acting up." As many asthmatics can readily testify, arthritis is not the only disease that is sensitive to changes in the weather. For some, any change in weather, including changes in barometric pressure, wind, or temperature, provokes asthma symptoms. For others, flare-ups occur under specific weather conditions—when it is too cold or too hot, too humid or too dry.

In addition to normal weather changes, smog and periods of heavy air pollution also spell trouble for many asthma patients. And as discussed in Chapter 7, events that coincide with seasonal changes, such as the rise of ragweed and other pollen in the late summer and fall or the flourishing of molds when it is damp and cool, also can trigger asthma.

Cold Air

As air travels through the upper part of the respiratory tract, it is warmed to body temperature. But when it is very cold outdoors, the nasal passages and upper part of the airways may not be capable of delivering warmed air to the lungs. When anyone gulps in a breath of cold air, the bronchial muscles will constrict to prevent the delicate lung tissue from being exposed to the potential damage from cold air. This response is likely to be even more pronounced in an asthmatic who has hypersensitive airways. And the more cold air that is drawn into the lungs, the more bronchospasm is likely to occur. Thus the person who may experience little or no difficulty walking down the street to catch a bus may experience considerable constriction and tightness if he or she attempts to run even a short distance. Any physical exertion results in faster and deeper breathing to meet the body's increased need for oxygen. Most asthmatics find that vigorous outdoor exercise when it is cold will bring on symptoms.

The best approach in dealing with cold-induced asthma is to avoid inhaling cold air as much as possible. First of all, avoid breathing through your mouth; the nasal passages are more efficient than the mouth and throat in warming air. To further warm the air, breath in through a ski mask, scarf, or handkerchief held over the nose. There also are special cold-weather masks which are available at pharmacies or medical supply stores. Taking a bronchodilator medication before going outdoors on a cold day also helps.

Pace yourself to avoid physical exertion in the cold. If you are worried about lack of exercise because you cannot engage in your usual outdoor activity, seek an indoor alternative. For example, instead of aerobic walking or jogging outdoors when it is cold, switch to an exercise bicycle or some other indoor physical activity. You may want to consider joining an exercise program at the Y or a health club during the cold months.

Wind

Next to the cold, wind is one of the most common weather-related asthma triggers. The wind itself may make breathing difficult. In addition, wind may carry extra asthma triggers, such as pollen or air pollutants. Anne Bronson, a thirty-two-year-old patient whom we met while visiting National Jewish, recalled her college days in southern California. "Cold weather always spells trouble for my asthma," she related, "so I thought that going to where it was always warm would be the best thing I could do. I had not counted on the effects of those hot, dry Santa Ana winds in California. They seemed to provoke my asthma almost as much as the cold. Luckily, they do not blow all the time, but when the winds came, I tried to stay indoors as much as possible."

Heat and Humidity

Some asthmatics find that their asthma improves during warm, humid weather, but for many others, such weather has the opposite effect. As noted earlier, high humidity fosters the growth of molds; but for some asthmatics, the humidity itself seems to be a trigger. Again, the best approach is to avoid exposure as much as possible. Staying indoors in an air-conditioned environment is often the best course. A room dehumidifier to remove excess moisture from the air also may be helpful.

Dry Air

There are some people with asthma who cannot tolerate overly dry air. For them, moving to the desert obviously is not the right solution to their asthma problem. A room humidifier may be needed to keep the air from becoming too dry—a humidity between 40 and 50 percent seems to be ideal for most patients. Care should be taken to make sure that the humidifier is cleaned frequently to prevent the growth of molds and other harmful microorganisms. Chemicals can be added to the water to retard the growth of molds, but these should not be a substitute for regular, thorough cleaning.

Smog and Air Pollution

Obviously, smog and air pollution are harmful even to normal, healthy lungs. For asthmatics and others with chronic lung disorders, they are doubly harmful. Most asthmatics find it more difficult to breathe during periods of high air pollution. There are some people with severe asthma who find they simply must move away from areas in which there is chronic smog or pollution. Tim Jackson is a case in point; he grew up near Missoula, Montana, where one would expect the Rocky Mountain air to be clean and pure. But the presence of several major pulp paper plants, combined with the valley setting and other atmospheric conditions, have made this an area of chronic smog. "No matter how hard I tried, I simply couldn't control my asthma," he recalled. "During a vacation trip to visit relatives in Oregon, my asthma became dramatically better, but when I went back to Missoula, I was back where I started. I finally realized that the air quality was the problem." Tim relocated to a coastal town in Oregon. The combination of unpolluted air, mild temperatures, and low pollen counts near the ocean have helped him bring his asthma under control.

Unfortunately, air pollution exists almost everywhere, and the problem cannot always be solved as easily as Tim's. Very often, in making such a move, a person will merely be trading one type of pollution for another. And, of course, it is not always possible to pick up stakes and move to avoid pollution.

Most pollution is man-made, and a growing number of localities are making efforts to reduce it. Missoula, for example, is attempting to restrict the use of wood-burning stoves, which add considerably to the air-quality problem. All of us can work with local environmental protection agencies to ensure that air-quality standards are observed. For anyone with asthma or other chronic lung disorders, living near an industrial area, refinery, smokestack, or other major source of air pollution should be avoided if at all possible. Staying indoors in an air-conditioned environment during periods of heavy pollution is advisable.

CHAPTER 13

Job-Related Asthma

With patience, diligence, and considerable detective work, most asthma patients can control their home environments to remove or minimize factors that provoke wheezing and other symptoms. However, dealing with asthma triggers in the workplace can be quite another story. Repeatedly, National Jewish patients recount the problems they have encountered in trying to overcome job-related asthma.

"It never occurred to me that my job was causing my asthma," an executive secretary explained. "I first developed asthma when I was twenty-six. My doctor had given me a number of skin tests, but had not found any particular substance that caused my wheezing. After I kept a diary of my symptoms, I realized that I invariably started feeling tight within an hour or so of going to work, and that I felt better on weekends and after I came home at night. My husband used to joke that I was simply allergic to my job, and I interpreted my problem to mean that my symptoms were due to some subconscious psychosomatic factors related to my job." Careful questioning and testing at National Jewish revealed that this young woman is particularly sensitive to chemicals used in the copying machine, which was next to her desk.

After she discussed the problem with her employer, the copy machine was moved to another room and others were assigned the job of copying. Her asthma control improved markedly.

Increasingly, there are cases of adults who develop asthma as a result of exposure to chemicals, fumes, or other substances in the workplace. It is estimated that of the 10 million or so asthmatics in this country, about 2 percent, or 200,000, have work-induced asthma. In an article in *Immunology & Allergy Practice* (Vol. 1, No. 1, 1979), Drs. C. Joe Anderson and Emil J. Bardana Jr. note: "The rapid proliferation of plastic and chemical compounds over the past several decades has dramatically increased the number of reactants which may induce work-related asthma."

Anyone whose symptoms appear or worsen while he or she is at work, and lessen or disappear while away from the workplace, should suspect job-related asthma. Occasionally a person will experience a delayed reaction, with the symptoms coming on during the night or even on the following morning. People who suffer nocturnal asthma should be asked whether the symptoms disappear when they are on vacation or have been away from the workplace for an extended period. If the problem returns, either gradually or all of a sudden, after returning to work, it is a good indication that the triggering factors are in the workplace.

Asthma often takes months or years to develop. Doctors at National Jewish frequently hear patients insist that they have worked with a particular substance without problems for years, so how could it suddenly produce asthma? Questioning often reveals that the patient may have had mild symptoms for long periods before the symptoms worsened and were recognized as asthma. Burning and tearing eyes, a scratchy, irritated throat, chronic coughing, and a runny nose are common early symptoms of a developing problem that may be ignored or attributed to persistent colds, allergies, or other disorders.

Tracking Down
Occupational Triggers

Identifying workplace substances that provoke asthma can be even more time-consuming and complicated than finding environmental triggers in the home or outdoors. Not uncommonly, employees will be unaware of what chemicals or other substances are present in the workplace. By law, all employees have the right to a list of the names of all chemicals to which they are exposed. Lists can be obtained from plant supervisors or union officials, or through the efforts of company nurses or physicians.

The nature of the job itself can be very revealing. Studies have found that large numbers of workers in chemical plants or the plastic industry, solderers in the electronics industry, platinum refiners, printers who work with color presses, and cotton carders suffer from work-induced asthma. In some instances, the potential triggers can be identified simply by the nature of the occupation. For example, carpenters and workers at sawmills that process Western red cedar require little investigation beyond their wood exposure. Molds, mites, and dust are the culprits for grain-elevator operators. Platinum salts are common asthma triggers among jewelers and photographers. (See Tables 19-22 for list of occupations and possible related asthma triggers.)

Table 19
High-Risk Occupations Dealing with Plastics, Chemicals, and Metals

Workers in the following fields should check with their employee health departments regarding specific agents that may cause asthma.

Adhesive industry	Jewelry industry
Bakeries	Lamination
Chemical industry	Meat wrapping
Clothing industry	Metallurgy and plating
Detergent industry	Paint manufacturing
Dialysis unit operation	Pharmaceuticals
Disinfectant industry	Photography
Dry cleaning	Plastics
Embalming	Printing
Food technology	Rubber industry
Fur trade	Shoe industry
Gardening and landscaping	Soldering
Grain elevator operation	
Hairdressing	Wood milling and preserving
Insulation industry (wiring, home, and others)	Word processing

(Adapted from *Immunology & Allergy Practice*, Vol. 1, No. 2, May/June 1979.)

Table 20

Causes of Work-Induced Asthma
Due to Wood and Vegetable Dusts

OCCUPATIONS	INDUSTRIAL EXPOSURES
Bakers	Flour (wheat proteins)
Carpet, felt manufacturers	Jute
Coffee workers	Green coffee beans
Farmers, grain elevator operators	Grain dust, grain weevil, grain mite, hops
Millers	Grain dust, grain weevil, grain mite
Oil and food industry workers	Castor beans, soybean flour and dust
Printers	Gum arabic, karaya, tragacanth
Rope, twine, and thread manufacturers	Flax, sisal
Textile workers	Cotton, flax, hemp
Tobacco workers	Tobacco
Trucking industry workers	Burlap sacks contaminated by coffee or castor bean dust, soybean dust, molds, or fungi
Wood workers	Wood dusts, molds

(From *Immunology & Allergy Practice*, Vol. 1, No. 2, May/June 1979)

Table 21
Causes of Work-Induced Asthma
Due to Pharmaceutical Agents

OCCUPATIONS	INDUSTRIAL EXPOSURES
Anesthesiologists	Enflurane
Antibiotic workers	Ampicillin, penicillin, spiramycin, sulfathiazole
Chemical plant workers	Phenylglycine acid chloride
Farmers	Spiramycin
Pharmacists	Pancreatic enzymes
Poultry food manufacturers	Amprolium hydrochloride
Veterinary and medical practitioners	Piperazine dihydrochloride, spiramycin

(From *Immunology & Allergy Practice,* Vol. 1, No. 2, May/June 1979)

Table 22
Causes of Work-Induced Asthma
Due to Substances of Animal Origin

OCCUPATIONS	INDUSTRIAL EXPOSURES
Animal handlers	Hair dander, mites, molds, small insects
Beekeepers, entymologists	Insect by-products, bee and insect toxins, hair chitin
Farmers	Animal dander, hair, and blood serum
Feather workers	Uncleaned feathers, mites

OCCUPATIONS	INDUSTRIAL EXPOSURES
Hairdressers	Human dander
Insecticide users	Insect by-products
Mushroom workers	Molds, fungi
Oyster workers	Marine organisms in oyster shells
Silkworm cutters	Silk hair, silk glue
Stockyard workers, taxidermists	Animal dander, hair, mites, molds, small insects

(From *Immunology & Allergy Practice,* Vol. 1, No. 2, May/June 1979.)

In many instances, likely offending substances will become apparent as a result of simply keeping a diary of contacts and symptoms. In some instances, the suspicion can then be confirmed by skin tests. More often, however, inhaled challenges are used to positively prove whether a particular substance is indeed producing the asthma symptoms. Sometimes tests can be done at the actual workplace, with the patient undergoing lung-function tests before and after work. Alternatively, a person may be instructed in how to use a peak-flow meter (see Chapter 4), so he or she can do self-testing at different periods throughout the workday. A drop of 20 percent in peak-flow readings suggests an environmental problem and the need for further testing. A rapid improvement in the peak-flow measurement after the taking of a bronchodilator medication indicates that the symptoms are due to asthma rather than some other lung disorder. A diary should be kept to see if changes in peak flow occur with specific tasks, at specific sites, or at specific times. Some types of occupational asthma are delayed, producing symptoms at night or in the early morning.

Any challenge testing using suspected asthma triggers must be done under careful medical supervision to prevent a severe, even life-threatening attack. The challenges should be conducted in a clinic, hospital, or doctor's office that is equipped to treat emergencies should they arise. Since responses may be immediate, delayed, or a combination of the two, it is usually necessary to wait up to eight hours or even longer before ruling out a substance as having no effect. A record of peak-flow measurements should be made repeatedly for twenty-four hours before and twenty-four hours after exposure.

Although this approach usually will identify workplace triggering factors, there are instances in which more time will be needed to determine for certain that the asthma is job-related. Sometimes the response to workplace triggers will be so erratic or, conversely, so constant that it is difficult to say whether the asthma is related to something in the home or at the job. A patient may be fine while at work and suffer delayed symptoms at night or in the early morning. There may not be any improvement on weekends or at other relatively brief periods away from work. If a doctor strongly suspects that something in the workplace is causing the asthma, the patient may be advised to stay away from it for a longer period to give the body a chance to recover without constant re-exposure. This may mean taking several weeks off from work. For example, a patient will undergo spirometric testing at the end of a workweek just before going on vacation. While away, the patient will be instructed to avoid any of the materials normally found at the workplace. He or she will be tested again at the end of the vacation to determine if there has been an improvement in lung function.

Complicating Factors

Treating occupational asthma is often complicated by the fact that there may be more than one mechanism that triggers a person's symptoms, even in instances in which a single substance is the cause. For example, a person may develop an IgE-mediated immune response to the substance. In addition, exposure to the substance may irritate the airways, thereby provoking inflammation and bronchospasm. The asthma may be accompanied by chronic bronchitis or emphysema, meaning that symptoms from these conditions are not reversible, and thus that only moderate improvement will be achieved with anti-asthma medications.

Common Job-Related Asthma Triggers

Specific occupations and related potential asthma triggers are listed in Tables 19–22. Of course, these are by no means the only workplace factors that can provoke asthma, and asthmatics should carefully consider the hazards that are inherent in a job when selecting a career or profession. A person with asthma who is highly sensitive to animal dander could expect to encounter major problems when working in a pet store, veterinarian's office or animal research laboratory. People bothered by tobacco smoke are likely to have problems in any public or private place where smoking is permitted. Surprisingly, some asthmatics fail to consider occupational exposure to asthma triggers when picking a career; more commonly, however, a person will develop occupational asthma as a result of exposure to workplace substances.

Occupational asthma usually refers to asthma related directly to the workplace. The person may have had mild childhood asthma, but not previously suffered from it as an adult. Or the problem may arise for the first time due to workplace exposure. The asthma sometimes comes on suddenly, shortly after starting a job, or it may develop gradually over a period of many years.

Dr. Richard Farr stresses that not all asthma attacks have

the same precipitating mechanism; this is particularly true in dealing with occupational asthma. Frequently, a person with job-related asthma will undergo extensive allergy testing, only to come up blank. In tracing asthma triggering factors, it is important to recognize that there are different types of asthma. Some factors may provoke the asthma by triggering an immune IgE-mediated response, and in these cases, allergies play an important role. Other asthmatics may experience attacks triggered by an inflammatory response to inhaling irritating gases, vapors, or particles. Still other attacks may stem from release of histamines or other natural mediators in response to a pharmacologic agent. Thus, a person who has no history of allergies and who tests negative on skin and blood tests may experience asthma attacks due to inhaling an irritating substance that causes inflammation of the airways, or exposure to a drug that increases the release of a variety of asthma mediators.

Treating Job-Related Asthma

The treatment of mild job-related asthma is similar to that of any asthma: eliminating or avoiding as many triggering factors as possible and using medication to prevent and reverse airway constriction. As a rule, allergy shots are not useful in treating occupational asthma. An exception may be animal-handlers' asthma, where the allergen is animal dander. In these cases, allergy shots may be beneficial. Otherwise, the offending substances are not as easily identified as dander, pollens, or other environmental allergens, and in many instances the asthma is not due to an allergy but to an airway irritation or other such mechanism. Perhaps the greatest difficulty in treating occupational asthma is in removing or minimizing the triggering factors. In some cases, the best solution may be to change jobs if there is no way that a triggering factor can be avoided.

In many industries, the offending substances endanger the health of all employees, not just those unfortunate enough to develop asthma. Although there is still much to be accomplished in reducing workplace exposure to harmful substances, increased efforts on the part of unions, employees, and employers are beginning to pay off. For example, a bacterial enzyme in some detergents was found to cause asthma. After this became known, the manufacturers ceased using it. In other instances of occupational asthma, improved ventilation systems, the use of protective masks, and changes in manufacturing processes are helping reduce exposure to airway irritants.

Of course, not all occupational asthma is confined to employees. A chemical or processing plant that spews irritating fumes, dusts, or other harmful pollutants into the environment may affect people who live, work, or play nearby. In recent decades, consumer action groups, unions, environmentalists, and others have been instrumental in enacting clean-air standards.

CHAPTER 14

Psychological Effects of Asthma

Throughout this book, we have repeatedly emphasized that, despite widespread notions to the contrary, asthma is not a disease with psychological causes. This does not mean, however, that there is not a strong psychological overlay or component in asthma. Very often, mental outlook and emotional factors determine how well a patient will be able to control his or her asthma. At National Jewish, psychological evaluation and counselling are important facets of the treatment.

Many factors are involved. For example, asthma is a chronic disease and the medications used to treat it can cause irritability and changes in body appearance. Thus, it is common for asthma patients to harbor strong feelings of anger and depression.

Anger

In the words of Dr. Richard Farr, former chairman of the Department of Medicine at National Jewish, "Asthma is a real downer of a disease and it can make a person very angry and hard to live with. Asthmatics don't necessarily start out angry, but after a few years, most will end up feeling frustrated, and at war with the world and everyone around them.

"We constantly hear about the sex drive or food drive, but very little about air drive," he explains. "Actually, this is the most basic and urgent drive of all. Without air, we can live only a very few minutes, whereas we can go days or even weeks without food. We hear that denial of sex can make a person angry and frustrated; this may be true, but it is not lethal. Anger is often a response to unconscious fear; in asthmatics, this is a fear of dying. If you want to see how even a very brief denial of air can lead to anger, put two friends in a swimming pool and tell them to play horse and rider. The horse swims underwater, with the rider astride his back. The two work out a signal that tells the rider when the horse needs to come up for air. Let the rider ignore that signal, and chances are the horse will come up fighting mad. An asthmatic has to live with unpredictable bouts of air hunger for life. One patient once said to me, 'Doctor, if you felt you were constantly breathing through a straw, you'd feel angry too.' "

In addition to the effects of the disease itself, many of the drugs used to treat asthma can cause feelings of jittery nerves, irritability, and mood swings. Many asthmatics have difficulty sleeping, which can increase the emotional toll.

Attitudes of family members, friends, and colleagues also can add to the asthmatic's feelings of anger and frustration. Anna Bronson, the National Jewish patient described earlier, told us how her growing up with asthma divided her family. "My older sister thought I was using my asthma to get attention, and my father tended to side with her. My mother became overly protective, and wouldn't let me run and play outdoors or do all the things my sister did. I became very jealous of my sister and vice versa—I thought she had all the fun and she was convinced that our mother cared more for me than her." Dr. Farr believes this is typical. "Show me a family in which one or more members have asthma and I will show you a family that is torn apart," he says. "The problems may not seem apparent, but probing will almost always bring out deep-seated resentments or feelings of guilt."

As Ms. Bronson grew older, she found that her difficulties were by no means confined to her family. "At school, the other kids thought I was the teachers' pet because I would be excused from chores and from activities like running around the track at gym time. I was absent a lot, so the teachers had to make exceptions for me. Even so, I always felt that I was behind everyone else." When Ms. Bronson started working, many of her colleagues thought she was malingering or using her asthma to gain special attention or favors. "I have always had difficulty forming real friendships," she says, "because I have never felt that I can give as much as I take. In fact, one of the most valuable aspects of my stay here has been the realization that I am not alone, and that there are many other people who share my frustrations and feelings of anger and inadequacy."

Denial

Denial is another common response to asthma—or to any frightening experience. From time to time, all of us have experienced situations in which we feel that by ignoring a symptom or a problem, it will simply go away. We all have said something like, "I'm not going to let this cold (backache, headache, etc.) get me down." And sometimes it seems to work. The ignored runny nose or back twinges or head pain disappears with time, and life continues on an even keel. But asthma does not work this way. The chest tightness, wheezing, and other symptoms will not go away simply by denying their existence or trying to "wait them out." All too often, this leads to a worsening of symptoms until a crisis stage necessitates yet another trip to the emergency room.

Anna Bronson recalled for us the consequences of her

denial of asthma warning signs. "It happened on the evening of our senior prom. At first, my mother had been reluctant to let me go, but she knew that I had been looking forward to this dance for months. On the morning of the big dance, I woke up feeling a bit tight, but I told myself it was only the excitement of knowing this was the big day. I got so caught up in doing my hair and nails and pressing my dress, that I even forgot to take my medication. By evening I really felt rocky, but I kept saying to myself, 'I'm going to this dance even if it kills me.' And it almost did. I think we had danced only a couple of dances before I was really having difficulty breathing. I had left my inhaler at home because it wouldn't fit in my tiny evening bag. I told my date I had to get some air for a few minutes and he walked outside with me. At first he didn't realize that I was in real trouble, but when I started gasping for breath he ran for one of the chaperones and luckily she knew about my asthma and got me to the emergency room. I ended up spending my prom night in the hospital, but that experience taught me once and for all that my asthma was not something I could wish away."

The patient is not the only one who experiences denial; quite often, parents think that their child will "tough it out" he or she can overcome an asthma attack. "We see this attitude more often in fathers than mothers," Dr. Strunk says. "Fathers want their children, especially sons, to be strong and tough. Very often, they interpret the asthma as a willful sign of weakness instead of an illness that requires treatment." This attitude stems in part from the erratic nature of asthma. A person may go for days or even weeks and months feeling perfectly fine, and then suddenly experience symptoms. Since the attack may be triggered by any of a number of diverse factors such as, for example, an emotional upset, a change in the weather, exposure to an allergen, or physical exertion— there may be a natural tendency to look upon it as an act of contrariness or an attention-getting device.

The very unpredictability of asthma often makes it easy

to deny, says Dr. Farr. "No one wants to think they are not in control of their lives," he explains. "Imagine what it must be like not being able to give a dinner party on Saturday night or have an outing with your children because you never know whether you are going to feel up to it." In this respect, asthma differs from many chronic diseases. A person with arthritis can be reasonably certain that if he or she takes medication and follows a treatment regimen, it will be possible to give the dinner party or go on the outing. In contrast, an asthmatic may be perfectly all right on the morning of the dinner party and then start experiencing symptoms just before the first guests arrive. "It is the uncertainty that can be so very difficult," Dr. Farr says, "and one of our main missions is to help people anticipate problems and take early preventive action. You can't do this if you are constantly denying there is a problem."

Using Asthma for Secondary Gain

There are asthmatics who do use their disease for secondary gain. "We often see this in troubled families," Dr. Farr explains, "where a child's asthma becomes a distraction on which the parents can focus to keep from confronting other underlying problems."

A common example involves the child who invariably suffers an attack when his or her parents quarrel. The parents stop fighting and focus their attention on the child's asthma. Unwittingly, the child is assuming the role of arbitrator of the parents' problems; but instead of confronting and solving whatever it is that is troubling their marriage, the parents' attention is shifted to the youngster's asthma. An important tip-off that this might be happening is the fact that the child's asthma gets better during a visit to Grandma or a summer away at camp.

"Not uncommonly, a child's asthma will improve dramatically shortly after arriving here without any real change in the treatment regimen," Dr. Strunk says. "In such instances, we have to probe to determine what there is about the home situation that promotes the asthma. Sometimes it will be a physical triggering factor, such as the presence of a dog or cat. But it also may be the emotional environment in which someone—the child or parents—are in some way benefiting from the asthma." In such instances, it is usually necessary to treat the entire family to bring about real improvement in the child's asthma.

Still another reason for denial may be rooted in apprehension about the need for certain treatments. "Many patients will do almost anything to avoid going on steroids," Dr. Farr explains, "because they know the long-term consequences of these drugs. So when a doctor says 'How are you doing?' they will deny they are having problems simply because they don't want to go on steroids." Pulmonary function tests will quickly tell a doctor whether the patient is, indeed, doing well or if there are problems that require more aggressive treatment. When caught in time, progressive asthma often can be brought under control by a short course of steroids, after which the patient is weaned off the drug to avoid the long-term adverse effects (see Chapter 16).

Discipline and Asthma

A person with asthma, especially a child, also may "use" the asthma to avoid discipline or unpleasant tasks. Behavior problems are not uncommon among asthmatic children, and very often the problem lies in the parents' reluctance to discipline them or to set limits for fear of provoking an attack. The child who starts wheezing when a parent says "no" or attempts to discipline him or her is a classic example of one who is using the disease for secondary gain. As noted by a National Jewish psychologist, it is not unusual for a person with a chronic disease to become manipulative. Parents need to recognize that even if discipline seems to provoke a child's wheezing, failure to set limits and teach proper behavior may create problems far more serious than the asthma itself.

At National Jewish, there is a special unit for children whose behavior and emotional problems are interfering with their asthma treatment and overall development. Common problems seen among these children include acting out, refusal to take medication as prescribed, and failure to achieve potential in school. Recognizing and treating the behavior and emotional problems often produces a dramatic improvement in asthma control. Again, it is important to emphasize that the psychological problems of these children did not cause their asthma, but, instead, exacerbate the condition and make treatment more difficult.

Role of Counselling

Many asthmatic people can overcome the psychological problems associated with their disease simply by recognizing them and talking them through with an appropriate person or persons. This may be a parent, spouse, doctor or therapist, or other asthmatic patients. "Finding a doctor who is both skilled in treating asthma and who will listen and really care is extremely important," Dr. Farr stresses. "Doctors have a natural tendency to want to 'fix' things, but asthma is not a disease that can be 'fixed'; it can be controlled, but not cured." In selecting a doctor, Dr. Farr suggests an initial interview in which the patient tries to assess how well the doctor is listening to the patient, and how interested the doctor really is in the patient's problems. "Treating asthma takes time, and much of the doctor's time should be spent just listening to what the patient is saying about how he or she feels. It is hard to do this in a ten-minute session in which most of the time is spent listening to the lungs and doing a quick lung-function test."

Group therapy with other asthmatics can be very helpful. Anna Bronson stressed this when she said, "I used to think I was the only person who felt the way I did, who had these experiences. Here I have found that there are thousands of others who have been down the very same road. Simply knowing I am not alone has been extraordinarily important. If others can cope and live normal lives with this disease, then so can I."

Family therapy also may be an important aspect of treatment, especially where a child is involved. Many parents are reluctant to turn to a family therapist because they feel this is a reflection upon their ability to be good parents. However, seeking family therapy does not imply failure or inadequacy; on the contrary, it can be an important step in the right direction.

It is important to realize that stress is a fact of life, and that it is not necessarily a negative one. The way in which we cope with stress determines whether it will become a major detrimental factor in our lives. Asthma produces stress and stress provokes asthma; still, this vicious cycle is far from unbreakable. As we have seen in this chapter, there are many ways of dealing with stress: denial, anger, delaying treatment, on the one hand; and communication, recognition, and other positive coping techniques on the other. Emotional difficulties are to be expected in living with any chronic disease, especially one like asthma. But they do not need to dominate life or to interfere with treatment.

CHAPTER 15

Sex and Asthma

To all of us, maintaining a close and loving relationship with a spouse or partner is one of life's most pleasurable and rewarding endeavors. And, of course, sex is a very important part of any love relationship. Unfortunately, for many people with asthma, sexual activity poses a special problem—one that patients and their partners are often reluctant to discuss with doctors, physical therapists, or others who may be able to help.

Many people with chronic diseases find that their sex lives suffer. Sadness, depression, insecurity, physical disability, medications, alcohol, and pain are but a few of the factors that interfere with sex. The asthmatic has a number of other problems to add to the list. Foremost is the fact that sexual activity, like any exercise, can provoke bronchospasm and a flare-up of symptoms. Obviously, the prospect of wheezing and the tension it creates will quickly dampen the sexual desire of both partners. For some, even kissing may inhibit breathing enough to cause apprehension and tightness.

In addition to the physical problems that may be encountered in lovemaking, an asthmatic may be overly self-conscious about physical changes such as weight gain, or bad breath due to chronic respiratory infections, and feel less attractive than previously. Of course, only some of the problems stem from the asthmatic; the spouse or other partner may avoid sex for fear of provoking symptoms.

Doctors at National Jewish realize that just because a patient or spouse does not bring up sex as a problem area, is no reason to believe such a problem does not, in fact, exist. Patients are given a very informative booklet, *Being Close,* that offers practical advice. In addition, physicians and others who are working with the patient and the family members attempt to bring this issue into the open.

"Many people have the idea that getting the right medication and controlling their symptoms are their major objectives in seeking treatment," Dr. Richard Farr observes. "Obviously, these are primary concerns, but the quality of life and relationships will have an important bearing on how well patients manage their asthma."

Importance of Communication

Patients are encouraged to discuss their problems and fears, with their partners as well as their doctors. Talking openly about feelings with your partner is a vital first step in paving the way for a more relaxed approach to sexual activity. Take, for example, shortness of breath during sex. In general, sexual intercourse requires no more exertion than climbing a flight of stairs or taking a brisk walk. If you can perform these other activities without shortness of breath, then sexual intercourse should not cause serious breathing problems. Still, understanding that shortness of breath during intercourse may be expected can ease anxiety. Moreover, by knowing what to expect, the partner with asthma can take preventive steps, such as using a bronchodilator before going to bed. If a person uses supplementary oxygen, increasing the flow may be advisable.

Communication the Key

Couples also should realize that sexual closeness entails more than having intercourse; indeed, intercourse need not always be the objective. Simply enjoying intimate times together—talking, listening, sharing, holding, caressing—is perhaps more important in a loving relationship than the sex act itself. The sexual nature of any relationship changes with time; striving for the "performance standards" of youth is both detrimental and disappointing. Some changes are a natural aspect of aging, and are unrelated to asthma. An older man may find that it takes longer to achieve an erection; an older woman may have diminished lubrication—eventually, all of us experience these changes, but they certainly do not herald the end of an active, satisfying sex life. Talking out these problems, both with each other and with a doctor or therapist who can provide specific guidance, is a major step in the right direction.

Still, broaching the subject of sex is often easier said than done. Many of us have problems when it comes to openly discussing sexual intimacy, even with our partners. Once you do break the ice you will likely discover that future discussions will become more comfortable and you will be well on your way to working out your own solutions. National Jewish therapists suggest that one way to begin might be to share reading material, such as this chapter with your partner. If you and your partner find that it is still too difficult to openly discuss your sexual relationship, a referral to a professional counselor may be in order.

Effects of Medications
and Other Disorders

As noted earlier, there is a long list of factors that can affect sexual function for anyone, with medications among those that are often overlooked. Many drugs can interfere with sexual desire and functioning. This side effect is not as common with the medications used to treat asthma as with others; but if a person is taking drugs for high blood pressure, or using antidepressants or tranquilizers, these may well cause reduced desire and, for men, difficulty in achieving erections. Alcohol also can decrease sexual ability and desire.

While the medications used to treat asthma usually do not affect sexual function, they may have an indirect influence. Steroids, for example, can cause changes in mood. Theophylline can cause feelings of shakiness, whereas bronchodilators can produce shakiness and increase the heartbeat. Such reactions can understandably detract from sexual desire. When taking any medication, always ask your doctor or pharmacist about possible side effects, including effects on sexual function.

Asthma, of course, is not the only disease that can interfere with sexual function. Diabetes is one of the most common causes of male impotence, which is often one of the first signs of the disease. For older women, menopause invariably means a thinning of vaginal tissue and reduced lubrication, which can lead to painful intercourse. Sometimes a nonprescription lubricating jelly or ointment is sufficient to overcome this problem; eventually, however, an estrogen cream or hormone replacement therapy may be needed. In any event, this is something that should be discussed with a doctor.

Practical Suggestions

There are many practical approaches a person can take to minimize the effects of asthma on sexual function. Daily exercise, for example, not only improves overall health and well-being, but increases physical stamina. And anything that increases stamina will reduce the likelihood of breathing problems during sexual activity.

Premedication with a bronchodilator also may help. The strategy is the same as premedication before exercise or any other activity that is likely to provoke bronchospasm.

Many couples are very conventional in their lovemaking techniques, overlooking the fact that certain positions may require greater effort from one partner or may be uncomfortable for a person with breathing difficulties. In this respect, couples should not hesitate to experiment in finding positions that are comfortable and pleasurable for both without placing undue strain on the asthmatic. For example, making love with both partners in a sitting position facilitates easier breathing. A side position is easier for a partner who needs to wear an oxygen apparatus. Having the woman astride the male partner conserves his energy. A position in which the woman is propped up with pillows and the man is kneeling over her eases all pressure from her chest, making it easier for her to breathe and also to use oxygen if needed. Sex is one area in which creativity and experimentation, with careful regard to the comfort and possible limitations of the partner, can pay off in increased pleasure and a closer overall relationship.

CHAPTER 16

Drugs to Treat Asthma

Heretofore, we have concentrated on describing what happens in asthma and how patients can go about minimizing its effects. At one time or another, most asthma patients will require more than preventive measures; they also will need drugs both to overcome an attack and to prevent or minimize future ones. Understanding how these drugs work, and how they should be used to gain the maximum benefit with the minimum risk of side effects, is a vital part of the self-management of this disease. Unfortunately, there are still many doctors who neglect to teach their patients the most effective methods of using their anti-asthma medications. "We constantly see this in the patients who come here," Dr. Reuben Cherniack told us. "We constantly encounter patients who have been taking inhaled medications improperly for years, and they are truly shocked to learn that there are better techniques that will provide faster and more effective relief of their symptoms."

The drugs used to treat asthma can be confusing even to the long-standing asthma patient, and can overwhelm anyone newly diagnosed with the disease. Questions that need to be answered include: What medication should I take during an attack? How soon should it be used? How many times should I take it? Do I need to take medication even when I am feeling well? Why use a nebulizer instead of a simple inhaler? Will these drugs make me fat or have other side effects? Is there anything I can do to prevent those side effects?

Ideally, the physician or the nurse will explain how and when to use each medication, as well as any equipment needed. But all too often a doctor or nurse's busy appointment schedule, or their lack of awareness of individual needs, may leave the patient confused as to how best to manage the asthma. Following are the major classes of drugs and how they are used in the prevention and treatment of asthma.

There are several different classes of drugs used to control asthma. Since these drugs have different mechanisms of action, they may be used alone or in combination, depending upon individual circumstances. The most common anti-asthma drugs prescribed in this country are the bronchodilators, which work by opening up the airways, making breathing easier. Aside from the injectable forms used to treat severe bronchospasm, aerosol use provides the fastest relief during an attack. In general, bronchodilators are prescribed both for daily use when a patient is feeling well and as a preventive measure before anticipated exposure to anything that might trigger an attack. They also are used to halt an asthma attack. National Jewish doctors teach patients to use their prescribed aerosol bronchodilator at the first sign of wheezing, chest tightness, or shortness of breath, or the onset of a coughing spell. Waiting until symptoms become worse may make it more difficult to effectively inhale the drug; or it may cause more medicine to be required, increasing the possibility of side effects.

The second most commonly prescribed family of drugs are the xanthines, with the theophylline preparations being the most familiar. Theophylline's mechanisms of action are not fully understood, but it is known that the drug opens the airways by relaxing the smooth muscles of the bronchi. Theophylline also makes the diaphragm more contractible and has been suggested to increase the clearance of mucus from the airways.

Some asthma medications are intended to prevent attacks rather than treat symptoms. Cromolyn sodium is the most common medication in this category. Cromolyn does not relieve bronchospasm; therefore, it should not be taken during an actual asthma attack.

Corticosteroids, which are powerful anti-inflammatory drugs derived from the adrenal steroid hormone, cortisol, are used when patients do not get sufficient relief from bronchodilators and other asthma medications. They are highly effective in reducing inflammation in the bronchial tubes, decreasing mucus secretions, and increasing the effectiveness of other medications. But steroids have many drawbacks, including a long list of side effects when used chronically.

Anticholinergic medications are still another class of drugs used to treat asthma, although they are not prescribed as often as bronchodilators, theophylline, and other medications. These drugs block the effects of acetylcholine, a neurotransmitter, thereby preventing tightening of the bronchial smooth muscles. They also reduce mucus secretion and coughing.

Other medications that may be prescribed to treat asthma include antihistamines and decongestants. Antibiotics, antacids, and nutritional supplements may also be added to the asthma patient's regimen to prevent or treat problems related to the disease.

Proper Techniques

National Jewish doctors stress the importance of using proper techniques in ensuring that asthma medications produce their desired results. The objective is to derive the maximum benefit from the smallest possible drug dosage.

Many National Jewish patients are surprised to learn that they have been using improper techniques to take medications—especially aerosols, or inhaled drugs—for years. No matter how powerful the medication, if it does not penetrate deep into the bronchioles it will not produce the desired effects. All asthma patients should ask their doctor, a nurse, or another qualified health professional to show them the proper way to take their asthma medication. At National Jewish, patients are taught how to use a nebulizer, which delivers a diluted amount of medication over a slightly longer period of time. This allows the drug to penetrate more deeply into the airways, reaching the smallest bronchioles. A metered-dose inhaler, or whiffer, may be easier to use than a nebulizer, but since it delivers a large amount of medication all at once it is not as effective. If the airways are badly obstructed, the concentrated drug dosage may produce side effects before the drug has fully penetrated the airways. By using a nebulizer, the patient can achieve maximum penetration of the drug with a minimum of adverse effects. Tables 23 through 27 describe proper methods of using inhaled medications. Following are more detailed descriptions of specific drugs, their uses, and their side effects.

Table 23

When to Use an Aerosol Medication

Take a full treatment as prescribed by your doctor:
- every night before going to bed.
- every morning when you wake up.
- at the prescribed frequency.
- when your chest begins to feel tight, or you develop coughing, wheezing, or shortness of breath.
- just before you undertake an activity (i.e., exercise) or are exposed to a substance that you know causes chest tightness, coughing, wheezing, or shortness of breath, such as cold air, cigarette smoke, dusty rooms, etc.

Call Your Doctor If:
- you need more than eight treatments in a day.
- your requirements for medicine (i.e., the number of treatments in a day) increases and this does not improve over one day.

Table 24

How to Use a Metered-Dose Nebulizer

1. Add the extender provided, such as a length of flex-tube or a spacer and a mouthpiece to the end of the nebulizer.
2. Follow the instructions of your doctor; or you may want to ask him or her about the following techniques, which are advised for adult patients by doctors at National Jewish:
3. a. Blow out a little air beyond the normal expiration.
   b. Put the mouthpiece into your mouth and close your lips around it.
   c. Squeeze the metered dose inhaler as you start the very slow inhalation.
   d. Take in a *very slow* maximum breath, *as if you were sipping hot soup.*
   e. When you can get no more air or medicine into your lungs, stop squeezing the metered-dose nebulizer and hold your breath as long as comfortably possible (up to ten seconds).
   f. Take the mouthpiece out of your mouth, let the air out, and wait for one minute.
   g. Wait a few minutes and take a second inhalation.

h. If the symptoms are not relieved, the dosage may be repeated *if* you are not experiencing the following side effects: (1) a "jittery" or jumpy feeling; (2) a noticeably faster heartbeat. Check with your doctor for further instructions.

Table 25
How to Use a Hand-Bulb Nebulizer

Preparing the Solution

1. Use a 1:1 solution unless directed otherwise by your physician. Put an equal amount of medication and saline or tap water into the nebulizer.

   This can now be left in the nebulizer. Do not worry if it changes in color; medication can be stored for up to twelve hours. Keep the remainder of the bottle of medication in the refrigerator.

2. Remove the plastic plugs. This allows air to enter the nebulizer during the treatment.

3. Add the extender provided such as a length of flex-tube and a mouthpiece to the end of the nebulizer.

4. Check the nebulizer by squeezing the bulb several times to see that a mist comes out of the mouthpiece.

5. a. Blow out a little air beyond the normal expiration.

   b. Put the mouthpiece into your mouth and close your lips around it.

   c. Begin to repeatedly squeeze the bulb of the nebulizer.

   d. Take in a *very slow* maximum breath, *as if you were sipping hot soup,* while repeatedly squeezing the bulb three or four times per inhalation.

   e. When you can get no more air or medicine into your lungs, stop squeezing the bulb and hold your breath as long as comfortably possible (up to ten seconds).

   f. Take the mouthpiece out of your mouth, let the air out, and wait for one minute. If you are still experiencing symptoms, the dosage may be repeated unless you are feeling jittery or experiencing an increased pulse rate. Call your doctor for further instructions if you are experiencing side effects from the medications and are still having symptoms.

When you will be away from home, pour the prescribed dose into the nebulizer and close the openings with corks so it can be carried in a pocket or purse. In addition, a five-inch corrugated tube and mouthpiece (essential for treatment) should be included, wrapped in a plastic bag to keep them clean.

Table 26

How to Use a Nebulizer with Y-Tube (Air Compressor-Driven)

Follow instructions for preparing the solution listed under Hand-Bulb Nebulizer.

---

1. Remove plastic plugs and add extender as for hand-bulb nebulizer.
2. Check the nebulizer by putting your finger over the Y-tube to see that a mist comes out of the mouthpiece.
3.a. Blow out a little air beyond the normal expiration.
   b. Put the mouthpiece into your mouth and close your lips around it.
   c. Put your finger over the Y-tube.
   d. Take in a *very slow* maximum breath, *as if you were sipping hot soup,* while keeping your finger over the Y-tube.
   e. When you can get no more air or medicine into your lungs, take your finger off the Y-tube and hold your breath to the count of ten.
   f. Take the mouthpiece out of your mouth, let the air out, breathe normally for one minute, and check for the indicators of sufficient medicine described in Tables 24 and 25.

Table 27
How to Clean Your Nebulizer

To prevent lung infection from a dirty nebulizer, use the following simple cleaning methods.

BEFORE EACH TREATMENT

1. Use a clean eyedropper or syringe to measure medications. Be careful not to touch the tip or you may contaminate it.

2. Replace bottle caps promptly and close tightly. Once medication bottles have been opened, store them in the refrigerator. Most medications can be kept out of the refrigerator for short periods of time.

AFTER EACH TREATMENT

1. Rinse nebulizer under a strong stream of warm water for thirty seconds.

2. Shake off excess moisture. Allow to air dry on a clean towel. Before storing your equipment you may want to dry the nebulizer by attaching it to your air compressor (if you have one) and blowing it dry.

MONDAY-WEDNESDAY-FRIDAY/OR EVERY OTHER DAY

1. Wash nebulizer completely with a mild dish soap and warm water.

2. Rinse thoroughly under running, warm tap water.

3. Completely immerse nebulizer and tubing, but not hand-bulb, for thirty minutes in a solution of one part white vinegar and two parts water. Discard vinegar after each use.

4. Rinse nebulizer thoroughly under running, warm tap water for one minute.

5. Allow to air dry on a clean towel.

6. Keep the nebulizer and eyedropper (or syringe) clean and dry. Store in a closed plastic bag.

7. Clean canister-type inhalers in the same manner.

Beta-2 Agonists

These drugs are bronchodilators and the most widely used asthma medications in this country. They are prescribed to both prevent and relieve acute asthma attacks by acting on beta-2 receptors to relax bronchial passages and slow the release of histamine from the mast cells. They also make cilia in the respiratory tree beat faster, clearing mucus from the lungs and making breathing easier.

Drugs in this category include epinephrine (Adrenalin), metaproterenol (Alupent), and albuterol (Ventolin) (see Table 28). These medications may be taken in pill or liquid form, by aerosol spray, or subcutaneous (under the skin) injection. When an asthma attack becomes severe enough to warrant a trip to the emergency room, subcutaneous epinephrine or terbutaline may be the drugs of choice.

Table 28
Commonly Prescribed Beta-2 Agonists

GENERIC NAME	BRAND NAME AND METHOD OF ADMINISTRATION		LENGTH OF ACTION
Epinephrine*	Adrenalin	subcutaneous injection	1–2 hours
	Sus-Phrine	same	4–8 hours
Isoetharine	Bronkometer	metered-dose inhaler	2–3 hours
	Bronkosol	solution for nebulizer	same
Metaproterenol	Alupent, Metaprel	metered-dose inhaler and solution for nebulizer	3–5 hours
	same	tablet or syrup	up to 4 hours

GENERIC NAME	BRAND NAME AND METHOD OF ADMINISTRATION		LENGTH OF ACTION
Albuterol	Proventil,		
	Ventolin	metered-dose inhaler	4–6 hours
	same	tablets	4–6 hours
Terbutaline	Brethine,	subcutaneous	
	Bricanyl	injection	4–6 hours
		metered-dose inhaler	4–6 hours
		tablets	4–6 hours

* Also available in nonprescription form

Different beta-2 agonists have varying effects on other body systems, depending on the receptors they act on. For example, epinephrine also works on beta-1 and alpha receptors; a few consequences of this are raising the blood pressure and heart rate, slowing release of insulin from the pancreas, and narrowing the arteries supplying the skin and kidneys. Because of these broad actions, epinephrine may be contraindicated for people with high blood pressure, diabetes, heart disease, and glaucoma. On the other hand, the newer beta-2 agonists such as albuterol and metaproterenol are more selective; they do not act on alpha receptors and have far less action on beta-1 receptors than older beta-2 agonists, potentially making them safer for patients with other health problems and producing fewer side effects. These drugs are also longer acting than epinephrine; the effects of inhaled albuterol last four to six hours, compared to thirty minutes for epinephrine.

The side effects most common to beta-2 agonists—increased heart rate, tremor, and shakiness—are also signals that aerosol forms of the drugs have penetrated into the lungs, and should not be a cause of alarm to patients. As with any drug therapy, patients who are taking medications for other conditions should tell their physicians so that adverse effects related to drug interactions may be avoided. For example, most antidepressant drugs increase the cardiovascular side effects of beta-2 agonists, while beta blockers such as propranolol (Inderal) decrease the bronchodilating effects. Patients should also notify their doctors of any new health problems so that any necessary medication changes can be made.

Theophylline

These commonly used medications belong to the same group as one of our most familiar dietary substances—caffeine. Drugs in this family include theophylline (Theo-Dur, Slo-phyllin, and others), aminophylline (Somophyllin), and oxtriphylline (Brondecon, Choledyl).

Theophylline is usually taken in pill or liquid form. In the emergency room, intravenous aminophylline (a chemical form of theophylline that is easier to dissolve in water) may be used if the attack is not relieved by epinephrine. Patients with chronic asthma often need to take theophylline regularly, even when they are feeling well, because the drugs work best when a constant level of medication is maintained in the blood. Oral theophylline, especially in slow-release forms, is not used to relieve symptoms of an asthma attack and should be used only according to the prescribed schedule.

The major drawback of these drugs is the narrow margin within which they are both safe and effective. For the majority of patients, a blood level between ten and twenty micrograms of drug per one milliliter of blood meets these criteria. Below this, the medication may not work; above this, it may have unpleasant or dangerous side effects. Adverse reactions include restlessness and/or nervousness, as well as headache, insomnia, nausea or vomiting, abdominal cramps, palpitations, irregular heart rhythms, rapid heart rate, and convulsions.

Many factors can increase or decrease the blood level of theophylline (see Table 29). Dosages are usually calculated according to pound (or kilogram) of body weight. Children, for example, metabolize theophylline faster than young and middle-aged adults and require a higher dose per pound of body weight; the elderly metabolize the drug more slowly and should receive a lower dose per pound of body weight. Because of these varying effects of theophylline metabolism, patients should notify their physicians of any medications taken for other conditions, and of current or new health problems and changes in diet. Often, patients who cannot tolerate an effective dose of a theophylline may have to take a beta-2 aerosol for better control.

Table 29

Factors Influencing Theophylline Blood Levels

THE FOLLOWING MAY INCREASE THEOPHYLLINE LEVELS:

    Diet rich in carbohydrates and low in protein

    Caffeine-rich products

    Congestive heart failure

    Severe viral infections, especially pneumonia

    Liver disease (e.g., cirrhosis and hepatitis) or liver inflammation

    Medications

        cimetidine (Tagamet)

        allopurinol (Zyloprim)

        erythromycin (Erythrocin and others)

        troleandomycin (Tao)

        propranolol (Inderal)

        phenytoin (Dilantin) (when it causes liver damage)

        methyldopa (Aldomet)

oral contraceptives
trivalent influenza vaccine
other drugs that have an adverse effect on the liver,
such as certain cancer chemotherapy agents

THE FOLLOWING MAY DECREASE THEOPHYLLINE LEVELS:

Diet high in protein and low in carbohydrates
Cigarette or marijuana use
Medications
barbiturates (e.g., phenobarbital)
carbamazepine (Tegretol)
phenytoin (Dilantin)
rifampin

Cromolyn Sodium

In contrast to bronchodilator drugs, which directly open
air passages, cromolyn sodium (the brand name is *Intal)*
works earlier in an allergic reaction to stabilize the mast cells
and prevent the release of histamine. Once used as a drug of
"last resort," the drug has come into its own and is often
prescribed as one of the primary medications for treating
chronic asthma.

Cromolyn sodium is particularly effective for allergy-induced asthma and for attacks triggered by exercise. It also
may be helpful for asthmatics who are exposed to triggering
agents in the work environment. It may take four to six
weeks after first starting cromolyn sodium before full benefit
is felt. The medication does not relieve bronchospasm during
an attack but once a patient has been taking the drug, it may
prevent exercise-related attacks if used several minutes before the activity. The drug may be taken as an inhaled powder, by metered-dose inhaler, or dissolved in water for use
with a nebulizer. For runny nose due to allergies, cromolyn is
available as a nasal spray (its brand name is *Nasalcrom).*

One of the main advantages of cromolyn is its safety. Most people suffer few or no side effects. Coughing and temporary spasm of the bronchial passages following inhalation of the powder are the most common adverse reactions. These may be eliminated by proper use of the Spinhaler device with Intal, changing to another form of medication such as the metered-dose inhaler or the nebulizer, or use of a beta-2 agonist shortly before using cromolyn. The usual dose is four times a day which may be reduced when symptoms are under control. If symptoms permit, patients should continue to use the medication during a cold or an asthma flare-up for the extra protection it provides. However, it is important to realize that cromolyn is not a bronchodilator and that other medications such as a beta agonist, theophylline, or steroids must be used to reverse an attack.

Anticholinergic Drugs

Atropine is the prototypic anticholinergic drug, but because of the narrow margin between an effective dose and one that induces unpleasant side effects, it is not as commonly prescribed as other medications to treat asthma. The Food and Drug Administration has recently approved another anticholinergic drug, ipratropium bromide or Atrovent, which has fewer side effects than atropine.

Side effects of atropine include a dry mouth, rapid heartbeat, palpitations, insomnia, tremor, dizziness, blurred vision, constipation, and urinary retention. Chewing sugarless gum or sucking on sugarless hard candies, or using a humidifier to keep air moist may relieve a dry mouth. Ipratropium bromide is not as readily absorbed as atropine, so it does not have as many systemic side effects. It does not produce tremor, and it is preferred over atropine for patients who have a chronic cough, bronchitis, or excessive sputum production.

Atropine should not be used by people with narrow-angle glaucoma, obstruction of the bladder, prostatic enlargement, and some forms of heart disease. The medication can also increase the adverse effects of anticholinergic drugs used to treat Parkinson's disease and other disorders, tricyclic antidepressants (for example, Tofranil or Elavil), and antihistamines.

Anticholinergic medications are taken as an aerosol, either in ready-to-use form or as a powder to be diluted in saline (salt-water) solution. The medication should be kept in light-resistant, airtight containers at room temperature to prevent deterioration. Since different nebulizers result in varying amounts of drug absorbed into the lungs, the physician should be notified of any change in equipment in order to adjust the dose accordingly.

Corticosteroids

Although steroid drugs are important in the treatment of asthma, many patients and physicians are reluctant to use them because of their long list of side effects (see Table 30, Side Effects of Steroid Drugs and How to Minimize Them). Many of the long-term problems associated with steroid use can be avoided, however, by making sure they are used properly. In general, this entails using high enough doses during an acute phase to reverse the asthma quickly, and then to wean the patient off the steroids to avoid chronic use. As stressed by National Jewish's Dr. Reuben Cherniack, "Steroids can be life-saving and certainly deserve a place in the treatment of asthma. But their usefulness is hampered by the fact that so many people—patients and physicians alike—do not use them properly."

Table 30

Side Effects of Steroid Drugs and How to Minimize Them

The following is only a partial list of possible adverse reactions, focusing on those which may be at least partially controlled by the patient. Keep in mind that many of these are reversible once the medication can be stopped.

SKIN

Acne	Cleanse skin thoroughly but gently with mild soap.
Tendency to bruise, thinning of skin	Avoid abrasive or irritating materials. Use care when walking, running.

GASTROINTESTINAL SYSTEM

Risk of ulcers	Take drug with food to minimize gastric irritation. Use antacids or other anti-ulcer medication as prescribed. Report signs of abdominal pain or bleeding, including dark, tarry stools, to physician.
Weight gain, increased appetite	Watch food intake to minimize increased weight. Emphasize low-calorie, high-fiber foods that satisfy increased appetite. Report increases of five or more pounds to physician. Certain steroids promote sodium and water retention more than others and may result in weight gain and swelling of ankles and feet.

HORMONAL

Osteoporosis	People at high risk should have regular measurements of bone density to avoid excess thinning and risk of fracture. Vitamin D and

calcium supplements and a regular exercise program help prevent steroid induced bone loss. Postmenopausal women should take estrogen replacement.

Diabetes

Patients with latent or current diabetes may become hyperglycemic and require increased doses of insulin or oral hypoglycemics. Dietary control of weight gain is important.

METABOLIC

Potassium deficiency

Add an oral supplement or good sources of potassium to diet (leafy green vegetables, whole grains, citrus fruit, and bananas). Report signs of deficiency (muscle twitching, cramps, or spasm) to physician.

Calcium deficiency

Include dairy products in diet and report signs of deficiency (muscle twitching, spasm, or cramps) to physician.

EYES

Cataracts, increased pressure within the eyeball

Report any vision changes promptly to physician. Patients who do not have symptoms should have vision exam every six to twelve months including slit lamp and tonometry (internal pressure) check.

IMMUNE SYSTEM

Increased risk of infection

See physician for infections that persist in spite of measures normally taken to combat them.

MENTAL/EMOTIONAL

Mood disturbances including euphoria, depression,

Be alert for mood swings and any environmental circumstances irritability and, rarely, psychosis

other than medication that may be causing them. Report severe or disabling symptoms to physician who may prescribe an antidepressant or change steroid dose.

Aerosol Preparations

Side effects of steroids can be minimized by taking them in small aerosol (or inhaled) dosages. Aerosol preparations, which include beclomethasone (Vanceril, Beclovent), triamcinolone (Azmacort), and flunisolide (Aerobid), entail lower steroid dosages than the oral forms. In addition, smaller amounts of the drug are absorbed into the circulation than with oral forms, another factor that reduces side effects. Inhaled steroids are often used to wean patients from oral forms. Aerosol preparations are also useful for patients who do not get sufficient relief from bronchodilators or other medications; for example, they may be prescribed to supplement beta-2 agonists. To enhance penetration deep into the lungs, they are best used fifteen minutes after an inhaled beta-2 agonist. Aerosol steroids have no value during a severe attack and should be taken only as directed by the physician.

The major side effect seen with aerosol preparations is the development of fungal infections in the throat. This can be minimized by using a spacer device to take the drugs, and also by rinsing out the mouth and gargling after use to remove traces of medication from the mouth and throat.

Oral Medications

Oral steroid drugs, used in treating a wide variety of disorders, are among the most powerful—and potentially troublesome—means to manage asthma. Although the drugs are formulated from synthetic steroids, they have the same powerful effects on almost every organ system as the actual hormone, cortisol. Their use requires careful planning by the physician to minimize adverse reactions both during therapy and if the drug is to be withdrawn.

When other asthma drugs have not been effective, the physician may put a patient on a two- to three-week trial period with an oral corticosteroid. If this produces results, the dose will be lowered to the minimum amount that produces relief. If there is no improvement within three weeks, the drug should be stopped.

Doctors at National Jewish have found that problems with steroids may be best prevented by administering an oral form in a relatively low dose together with an aerosol in a higher dose. For acute flare-ups, high oral doses may be given for several days and then rapidly tapered back to a maintenance dose. Intravenous corticosteroids may also be used in the treatment of severe, progressive bronchospasm that does not respond to bronchodilators.

In addition to the amount of the drug and the method by which it is taken, the schedule of administration and diet also have an influence on the development of adverse reactions. Taking the drug on alternate days is the safest method; a single daily dose is the next safest schedule, and divided daily doses the least safe. National Jewish doctors stress that oral steroids should not be taken more than once a day on a long-term basis. Taking the medication early in the morning most closely resembles the body's natural secretion of cortisol. Corticosteroids, to different degrees, also produce reactions related to aldosterone, an adrenal hormone that regulates salt and water balance. For this reason many physicians advise patients, especially those with heart disease, to follow a low-salt diet.

Steroid Withdrawal

The body's endocrine system is extraordinarily sensitive to even minute changes in hormonal levels. When a person takes in extra steroids in the form of medication, the adrenal glands reduce their normal production of cortisol hormone. Oral steroids taken for two to four weeks or longer—physicians may differ as to duration and dose level—make the adrenals sluggish and may result in cortisol deficiency if the medication is discontinued suddenly or if some physical stress increases hormone requirements. Warning signs include nausea and vomiting, lack of appetite, lethargy, headache, fever, joint and muscle pain and stiffness. To prevent this deficiency, known as corticosteroid withdrawal syndrome, the physician will plan a tapering schedule based on the specific medication, length of time taken, size of dose, and other individualized factors. Patients should *never* abruptly stop taking oral steroids. In addition, stresses such as illness, viral infection, upcoming surgery, or a flare-up of asthma should be reported so that any necessary dose adjustments can be made.

As with any illness requiring drug therapy, asthma patients who are being considered for steroids should report any other health problems. Potential contraindications to oral corticosteroids include diabetes, hypertension, peptic ulcer, diverticulitis, and osteoporosis.

Supplementary Medications

Antihistamines and Decongestants

Asthma patients who suffer from runny nose, sneezing, or other hay fever symptoms may also be placed on an antihistamine or decongestant if congestion is the problem. Many of these drugs are available without a prescription and it may be tempting for the individual to "self-medicate" without mentioning additional drug use to the physician. Patients should remember that virtually all drugs have side effects of their own as well as interactions with other medications. For instance, the decongestant pseudoephedrine (Sudafed, Actifed, and others) belongs to the same chemical family as epinephrine and metaprotenerol; patients taking two of these drugs may have increased side effects from their combined actions. The antihistamine diphenhydramine (Benadryl) is also an anticholinergic drug and may exaggerate the adverse effects of atropine. Always check with your doctor as to the safety of adding a nonprescription drug to current medications.

Common side effects of antihistamines are drowsiness or, conversely, excitability; common side effects of decongestants are dry mouth, insomnia, tremors, and restlessness.

Drugs Used with Corticosteroids

Vitamin or mineral supplements may be prescribed for patients on oral corticosteroids to prevent osteoporosis (vitamin D and calcium) and disturbances in body chemistry (potassium supplements). Although these are given to prevent deficiencies, patients should also learn to recognize some of the more common signs of over-supplementation:

Calcium: loss of appetite, weakness, nausea and/or vomiting, abdominal pain, constipation, and increased need to urinate. The elderly, and people with kidney stones or other kidney diseases may be more vulnerable to calcium excess.

Vitamin D: same as for calcium. Vitamin D increases the body's absorption of calcium. Patients with impaired kidney function or sarcoidosis may be especially vulnerable.

Potassium: nausea and/or vomiting, abdominal pain or

bloating, diarrhea. Patients with kidney or heart disease may be especially affected.

Patients who have heartburn due to hiatus hernia or who are at risk for ulcers may be told to take antacids that neutralize stomach acid secretions, or medications that selectively block histamine receptors in the gastrointestinal tract, reducing acid secretion. Antacids usually contain aluminum hydroxide alone (Amphogel) or in combination with a magnesium compound (Gaviscon, Maalox), and an antiflatulent simethicone (Maalox Plus, Gelusil). Although antacids generally have few side effects, patients should keep in mind the following:

- Aluminum hydroxide alone can cause constipation. Ask your doctor if you can switch to a combination antacid if this occurs.

- Sodium contained in some antacids may promote water retention in patients on corticosteroids. Check the label before buying.

- Take antacids only as directed by your physician. Antacid use may be contraindicated in patients with kidney disease.

- Most antacids decrease the absorption of the antibiotic tetracycline and the anti-ulcer drug cimetidine (Tagamet), and neither should be taken with antacids.

Cimetidine or ranitidine, which are histamine-blocking medications, may be prescribed for asthma patients with a history of peptic ulcers or inflammation of the stomach or esophagus who must take oral corticosteroids. Common side effects of cimetidine include mild diarrhea, dizziness, and rash. Headache is the most common side effect of ranitidine. Cimetidine may increase theophylline levels in the bloodstream, but ranitidine does not seem to have this effect.

Medications to Prevent
Respiratory Infections

The hyperreactive airways that characterize asthma make it particularly important for patients to avoid respiratory infections. Yearly influenza vaccines are a must, and adults also should be immunized against pneumococcal pneumonia. For those who cannot take flu shots—either because of an allergy to eggs or because they already have the flu or a cold—amantadine (Symmetrel) can both prevent and alleviate respiratory symptoms due to type A influenza virus.

Symmetrel, which is also used to treat Parkinson's disease, is typically taken for ten days following exposure to the type A virus or as soon as virus symptoms begin, and for two to four days after they disappear. There is no evidence that the medication works against flu viruses other than influenza type A.

The most common side effects of Symmetrel are mental depression, psychosis, congestive heart failure, and dizziness or fainting due to orthostatic hypotension, a temporary drop in blood pressure when changing to a standing position. Symmetrel also increases the side effects of atropine and other anticholinergic drugs.

Antibiotics

Some doctors recommend that asthmatic patients take antibiotics at the first sign of acute respiratory infection, but National Jewish doctors do not follow this procedure, especially for children. Before taking an antibiotic, it should be confirmed that the problem involves bacteria. Sometimes this can be judged from the nature of symptoms, such as fever or a change in the amount, color, or consistency of the sputum. In other instances, a culture may be needed. If a bacterial infection is confirmed, an antibiotic appropriate for that microorganism should be prescribed. More commonly, the respiratory infection will be caused by a virus; in these cases, taking an antibiotic will not help and the patient incurs both the risk of side effects from the medication and the additional cost of a drug that is not indicated.

If an antibiotic is prescribed, the patient should take it for the entire course of treatment, even if symptoms improve after a day or two. Although the symptoms may disappear shortly after taking the drug, this does not necessarily mean that all of the causative bacteria have been eliminated. Stopping the drug too soon may leave behind surviving bacteria capable of producing strains that are resistant to the antibiotic. The patient also will be vulnerable to reinfection. If symptoms are not relieved after one to two days, the patient should contact the physician again, since this may be a sign that the drug is not effective against the bacteria involved.

Medications to Avoid

Combination Drugs

Some asthma medications, available both with and without prescription, contain a combination of active ingredients. Examples are Marax (ephedrine, theophylline, and hydroxyzine, a tranquilizer); Bronkotabs (ephedrine, theophylline, phenobarbital, and guaifenesin, an expectorant); and Tedral (ephedrine, theophylline, and phenobarbital). Most physicians recommend that their patients avoid these preparations because the ingredients cannot be tailored to individual needs and pose a greater risk of side effects due to the drug interactions.

Nonprescription drugs, whether in combination or as single ingredients, are usually not recommended by physicians; and many patients have the mistaken perception that they are not "serious" medications and do not need to be mentioned to the physician. For example, Medihaler-EPI and Primatene Mist contain epinephrine, a beta-2 agonist with widespread effects on many body systems. The easy availability of over-the-counter medications add to the potential for abuse in the uninformed patient.

Drugs Affecting Respiratory Function

The following drugs may either trigger asthma attacks or otherwise impair breathing:

Aspirin

People with extrinsic asthma have a higher incidence of reactions to aspirin than the general population. A 1970 study by Dr. Richard Farr found that 20 percent of adults admitted to National Jewish with severe asthma could not tolerate aspirin. Normal doses can trigger an asthma attack as late as three hours after ingestion. Those who are sensitive to aspirin may also react to indomethacin (Indocin) and other nonsteroidal anti-inflammatory drugs, including the nonprescription dosages of ibuprofen (Motrin, Advil, and others) that are often used to treat arthritis, menstrual cramps, headaches, and other pain syndromes. The problem is more common among adults; children under the age of ten usually do not react to aspirin.

Central Nervous System Depressants

Sedatives and narcotics often affect respiratory control centers in the brain and may impair breathing and coughing. Patients with extrinsic asthma may be hypersensitive to the barbiturate phenobarbital, used as a sedative and anticonvulsant but also found in drugs used to treat asthma (Bronkolixir, Bronkotabs, Isuprel HCL Compound Elixir).

Acetylcysteine (Mucomyst)

This drug is used to break up mucus secretions in patients with chronic lung disease and those with cystic fibrosis, and patients receiving general anesthesia. Paradoxically—and unpredictably—it can increase airway obstruction. Asthmatics who have taken this inhaled drug with no previous adverse reactions may develop them; conversely, those who have had a previous reaction may be able to tolerate the medication at a later date.

Propranolol (Inderal) and Other Beta-Blocking Drugs

Used to treat hypertension, angina, and irregular heart rhythms, these drugs can cause bronchospasm and should generally be avoided. The same is true of timolol maleate (Timoptic), a beta-blocking drug in the form of eyedrops used to treat glaucoma. Recent studies have found that these eyedrops can cause severe airway obstruction in some asthmatics.

Other Considerations

Every patient with asthma is different, and drug therapy must be carefully individualized according to individual needs. This may entail trying several drug regimens before arriving at one that works best for a particular person. Moreover needs may change with time or under different circumstances. For example, a person who does well with minimal drugs during most of the year may have a sudden flare-up during hay fever season or when the weather turns cold, and require different or additional medications.

Asthma is a chronic disease that often requires frequent visits to a physician. Maintaining good communication with the treating physician is important, especially for a patient with severe asthma. Many patients hesitate to call their doctor early in the course of an attack, not wanting to bother him or her with what may be a trivial problem. This can be a mistake, because the earlier a flare-up is treated with the appropriate medication, the less likely it is to progress to a serious or life-threatening episode.

CHAPTER 17

Breathing Techniques

Most of us breathe in and out tens of thousands of times each day without a second thought. Unfortunately, asthmatics do not have this luxury. For any patient with chronic lung disease, the objective is to breathe in enough air to provide adequate oxygen for the entire body, and to exhale carbon dioxide. In emphysema and some types of severe asthma, breathing techniques can be very important. Patients at National Jewish Center are taught the most effective ways of breathing, and many are instructed in specific breathing retraining exercises. Following are the National Jewish Center's guidelines for proper breathing techniques. At first, it may require a conscious effort to breathe this way, but, with practice, the technique should become automatic.

- Breathe in through the nose slowly and smoothly; pause and then pucker the lips as if whistling and let the air fall out slowly through pursed lips.

- Use the diaphragm and the pursed-lip technique to slow down breathing so that more air can move in and out of the lungs, while keeping small airways from closing down and trapping stale air.

- The rate of normal breathing should be about ten to fifteen breaths per minute.

- Synchronize this breathing with activity: Inhale while extending or straightening the trunk, lifting the arms up, or moving the arms away from the body. Exhale when flexing or bending the trunk or bringing the arms toward the body.

Retraining Exercises

People with poor muscle conditioning often require retraining exercises. Here are the ones taught at National Jewish, which should be practiced 10 to 15 minutes daily except when the patient is short of breath or feeling sick.

- Begin while sitting on a chair or something sturdy.

- With arms relaxed and hanging at the sides, raise your shoulders toward the ears, and then relax.

- Bend your head forward, chin on chest, then lift the head upward to look at the ceiling.

- Turn the head to alternate sides.

- Turn the head in a circling motion.

- Swing arms forward and then relax.

- Stretch your arms sideways to a position above the head while breathing in.

- Lower the arms while breathing out. (Some people may need to take two or three breaths while raising their arms.)

- Bend the elbows with fingertips on the shoulders, and circle the elbows forward, up, back, and down.

Diaphragmatic Breathing

Using the diaphragm increases breathing efficiency. Practice the following every few hours, resting after three or four breaths if you feel lightheaded:

1. Front expansion

- Inhale slowly through your nose while your stomach expands outward.
- Exhale slowly through pursed lips while the stomach draws inward. To test if your technique is correct, place one hand over the stomach to feel it move and the other over the upper chest to keep movement at a minimum.

2. Lower side expansion

- Breathe in slowly through your nose and allow your ribs to expand outward.
- Breathe out slowly through pursed lips, allowing the ribs to move inward. To check, place hands on your sides at the base of the ribs to check expansion.

Breathing Control Exercises

The following should be practiced during periods when breathing is difficult.

Lying Down

- Lean back against pillows or some other support, at whatever angle is most comfortable.

- An alternative is lying on your side and making a slope with three or four pillows, placing an extra pillow to fill the gap between waist and armpit. Lie high up on these pillows, with the whole of the side supported and the shoulder underneath the top pillow.

Sitting

- Sit in a comfortable chair in front of a table. Place pillows on the table and lean forward from the hips with a straight back, resting your head, shoulders, and arms on the pillows. The arms should be lying loosely on the table, while the shoulders and upper part of the chest rest against the pillows.

- Sit and lean forward with a straight back while resting your forearms on your thighs with the wrists relaxed.

Standing

- Lean forward from the hips onto something of the required height. Your back should be straight, arms spread well apart, and your head should rest on your hands.

- Lean the lower half of your back against a wall, with the feet placed about twelve inches away from the wall. The shoulders should be relaxed, the arms hanging loosely by the side.

Coughing

Coughing is one of the most important of the lungs' defenses. These drawings show how productive coughing helps loosen a mass of sputum and expel it from the body.

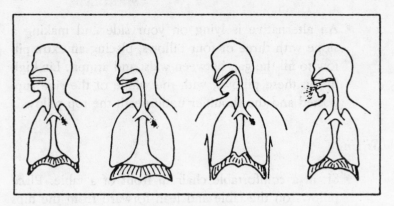

Figure 7

In the first drawing, the mass of sputum is seen near the bronchus (see Figure 7). In the second drawing a deep breath is pulled in. The diaphragm pushes up to increase the pressure inside the lungs, as shown in the third drawing. During the cough, illustrated in the last drawing, the epiglottis opens suddenly and the pressurized air is forced out of the lungs, shaking loose the sputum in the process and forcefully expelling it.

Postural Drainage

The basic idea of postural drainage is to assume a position that makes it easier for mucus and other secretions to flow out of the lungs. There are four basic positions for postural drainage, which are illustrated in the accompanying drawings (Figures 8–11). Each position should be maintained for at least ten minutes. During this time, breathe slowly and deeply through the nose, which promotes the use of the lower intercostal muscles (mouth breathing encourages the use of the upper intercostal and accessory muscles). While in the postural drainage positions, cough up as much mucus as you can every two or three minutes. Take in as much air as you can and give three sharp coughs before breathing in again. This is less fatiguing and will produce more sputum. Gravity and coughing will facilitate the flow of sputum.

Even more can be produced by having a companion clap the patient's chest over the appropriate lobes with the hand cupped to loosen the mucus. For clapping, the wrists should be loose while the arms, elbows, and shoulders should be extended but not rigid. The person clapping should place a towel over the patient's chest so that the impact of the cupped hand is firm but not painful. The clapping should be followed by a vibrating movement, in which the assistant places his or her hands one on top of the other with the palms down and the bottom palm resting on the same area, and then vibrates the area where the clapping was just performed. The clapping should be done for one minute and the vibration for three or four repetitions in each position.

The patient should drink something warm a half hour before the draining procedure, and take an inhaled treatment of bronchodilators, mist, or both before beginning.

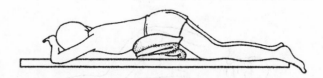

Figure 8
POSTURAL DRAINAGE—POSITION 1

This position drains the lower back segments.
Assume a position lying face down with the hips elevated 18 to 20 inches on a stack of pillows. Cough according to instructions. If someone is available to clap, this should be done from below the shoulder blade to approximately 3 inches above the bottom of the ribs, but not over the backbone or kidney.

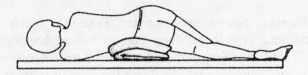

Figure 9
POSTURAL DRAINAGE—POSITION 2

This position drains the lower right lung segments.
Shift your body so that you are lying on your left side with your hips elevated 18 to 20 inches. Cough according to instructions. Clap over the middle portion of the side of the chest.

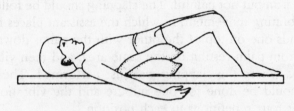

Figure 10
POSTURAL DRAINAGE—POSITION 3

This position drains the lower front lung segments.
Assume a position lying on your back with the hips elevated 18 to 20 inches. Cough according to instructions. Clap from below the nipple line to the bottom of the ribs, but not over the stomach.

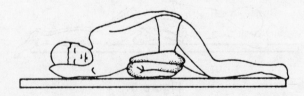

Figure 11
POSTURAL DRAINAGE—POSITION 4

This position drains the lower left lung segments.
Assume a position lying on your right side with the hips elevated 18 to 20 inches. Cough according to instructions. Clapping should be done over the middle portion of the side of the chest.

Oxygen Therapy

Most asthmatic patients do not require oxygen therapy except in emergency situations. But people with severe or chronic asthma, as well as patients with emphysema, severe bronchitis, and other lung disorders that leave them constantly short of oxygen will benefit from supplemental oxygen. When oxygen supplies are chronically low, the heart must work harder to try to supply enough oxygen to the body's cells. Eventually, the heart becomes enlarged and cannot work as efficently. Supplemental oxygen can prevent this from occurring, or can help prevent further heart damage.

If supplemental oxygen is needed, your doctor will determine the dosage and give detailed instructions as to how it should be used. It is important not to alter the dosage of oxygen except with a doctor's approval. Both too much and too little oxygen can be detrimental.

Types of Oxygen Systems

There are three basic types of oxygen systems. In a *compressed gas* system, the oxygen is compressed into steel or aluminum cylinders, which prevents leakage of the gas into the room. The units are portable—the steel ones weigh about seventeen pounds, the aluminum, thirteen pounds. Each provide about five hours of oxygen at two liters per minute.

In a *liquid* system, the oxygen is cooled and pressurized to its liquid form and placed in a thermos-type container called a reservoir. As the compressed liquid oxygen is decompressed, gaseous oxygen is formed that is provided for the patient through a breathing apparatus. The portable unit weighs eleven pounds and provides about nine hours of oxygen at two liters per minute.

The *oxygen concentrator* device works on the principle of

pumping air through a separating unit containing a sieve material that retains the nitrogen content of the air and permits the oxygen to be separated and concentrated into a reservoir for breathing. The unit weighs forty-five pounds, and provides about 95 percent oxygen at one liter per minute and about 75 percent oxygen at four liters per minute. The supply is endless so long as there is a battery or electrical outlet to provide power.

CHAPTER 18

Total Rehabilitation

Rehabilitation is an integral part of the overall treatment program at National Jewish. Almost from the time a patient checks in, National Jewish doctors, social workers, psychologists, exercise therapists and others go to work planning rehabilitation and discharge. The ultimate goal is both to bring the asthma under control and to help the patient lead as unrestricted a life as possible.

In earlier chapters, we discussed specific steps patients and their families can take to identify and remove or minimize environmental and other factors that provoke asthma attacks. Learning how to reduce the number and severity of asthma attacks obviously is a vital first step in the rehabilitation process. The same is true of exercise—as noted earlier, many asthmatics experience symptoms when they exercise, and, understandably, restrict physical activity to avoid provoking an attack. This sedentary life-style further reduces their tolerance to exercise; and the less the person exercises, the more intolerant to exercise he or she becomes. Thus, exercise training is an integral part of the rehabilitation process. (See Chapter 10 for a more detailed discussion.)

Energy Management

Most people go about their daily routines without ever giving a thought to how much energy certain tasks demand. Unfortunately, many asthmatics do not have this luxury. Routine tasks like taking a shower, grocery shopping, walking to the corner to buy a newspaper, and climbing two or three flights of stairs to reach a classroom can be exhausting endeavors that provoke wheezing and shortness of breath. Although most asthma patients can hold a job, go to school, and perform the day-to-day tasks demanded of them, many must pace themselves to avoid symptoms. At National Jewish, patients are taught how to analyze their individual situations and recognize ways in which they can conserve energy.

Since patients who come to the National Jewish Center suffer from asthma that is more severe than average, many are unable to hold jobs, go to school, or carry on normal daily routines. Although these patients may be unable to pursue a former line of work, there may be other jobs for which they are suited. Identifying the interests, aptitudes, skills, and resources that will help even severely disabled patients become more active is an integral part of formulating overall treatment goals for individual patients.

"Being afraid of an asthma attack, or becoming short of breath, may cramp your life-style so that you don't do the same things you used to enjoy," patients are told in their National Jewish notebook. "Gradually, without work, without a sense of independence, one may start to feel sluggish, turned off, and depressed." To reverse the cycle, the patients are taught how to more efficiently organize their days and allocate their energy. As a beginning, they are asked to keep careful records of what they do in a typical day. (See Table 31, My Daily Routine.) The idea is to apply the techniques of effective business management to personal lives. "In many

Table 31
MY DAILY ROUTINE

Daytime	Evening
5:00 a.m.	5:00 p.m.
6:00 a.m.	6:00 p.m.
7:00 a.m.	7:00 p.m.
8:00 a.m.	8:00 p.m.
9:00 a.m.	9:00 p.m.
10:00 a.m.	10:00 p.m.
11:00 a.m.	11:00 p.m.
12:00 Noon	12:00 Midnight
1:00 p.m.	1:00 a.m.
2:00 p.m.	2:00 a.m.
3:00 p.m.	3:00 a.m.
4:00 p.m.	4:00 a.m.

ways, the management of your life, your work, and personal affairs is like that of a business," the center's booklet explains. "Principles of good organization, planning, delegating responsibilities, and scheduling skillfully may make an enormous difference in the quality of life that you will live."

To see how this is applied to everyday routines, National Jewish rehabilitation experts take patients through an exercise in grocery shopping. "It can be very demoralizing for a person with asthma to have to depend upon others for help in so many routine tasks," one of the National Jewish therapists explains. This was reiterated by Susan Barclay, the young mother of three whose asthma had become increasingly disabling in recent years. "Waiting for someone to take you to the grocery store because you have difficulty loading and unloading the bags is time-consuming and humiliating," she recalls. "So was having to ask others to fill in when it was my turn to car-pool the kids to after-school classes. My children never complained, but I felt like I was letting them down."

Many of the suggestions for more effective energy management came as eye-openers to Susan. "When I first read the list, I thought: 'These are all so obvious.' But then I realized that even so, most had not occurred to me."

Specific suggestions include:

- Buy staples in sizes you can handle easily.

- Instead of carrying groceries, laundry, or other heavy objects in your arms, use a grocery cart that rolls easily on wheels. Heavy books can be carried in a satchel-type bag or knapsack that has shoulder straps. Suitcases with wheels and a pull strap are available, or can be pulled along on wheeled carts.

- Ask that groceries be sacked lightly to avoid lifting heavy bags in and out of a car. Have perishables that need refrigeration packed separately. This way, you can load them in your shopping cart and take them into the house immediately and put them away. If you feel tired, you can rest before getting the remaining bags without worrying that ice cream is melting or meat is spoiling.

- If a complete shopping trip is too tiring, have someone else shop monthly for heavy items that can be bought in bulk, such as laundry soap.

- In storing groceries and other items, place the ones that you use most often in easy reaching range without the need to stretch upward or bend over. Put items you will use first up front, so you are not constantly moving things from front to back. Lazy Susans can be used in cupboards and refrigerators to make it easier to move items.

Organize Work Centers

- Arrange your kitchen and storage areas so that items are near their point of use. For example, have a can-opener near the canned goods, and store vegetables near the vegetable preparation area.

- Set up a baking center, so that dry ingredients, mixer, mixing bowls, and measures are all within a small radius to eliminate unnecessary steps.

- Leave heavy appliances and utensils that are used frequently out on a counter or stove top.

- When starting a task, such as preparing a meal, gather all the equipment and materials together in the beginning to save extra steps and make for more efficient time management.

- When baking, have a sinkful of soapy water into which dirty utensils can be put immediately to pre-soak to save on later cleanup and also to avoid clutter as you work.

Other Energy-Saving Tips

- Use assembly-line principles to save unnecessary steps. For example, when preparing a meal, use a wheeled cart to move the items during the various processing steps.

- Use a cart to wheel cleaning supplies from room to room, thus eliminating the strain of carrying them and going back and forth. The same method can be used to put away clean clothes after doing the laundry.

- Work from easy heights. For example, using a dustpan with a long handle eliminates bending. When possible, sit down to do tasks like ironing, folding clothes, and paring vegetables.

- Whenever possible, utilize labor-saving devices. Perhaps your mother scrubbed the floor on her hands and knees and used a rug-beater to clean carpets. But modern electric floor cleaners and vacuums are even more effective and require a lot less elbow grease.

- Assign chores to other family members. You don't have to do it all. Giving others specific responsibilities eases the burden on you, fosters feelings of responsibility in children, and lets your family know where their help is most needed.

- REST WHEN YOU FEEL TIRED. Many asthmatics make the mistake of thinking, "I'll just finish this job before sitting down," even when they feel a tightening and the onset of other symptoms. Whenever you attempt a task that you know is going to be taxing or take a long time, plan rest breaks and *take* them. If this is difficult for you to do, create a "break center" with a comfortable chair and some reading or handwork you can do so you will not feel you are "wasting" your time.

Although the preceding lists apply mostly to housekeeping tasks, the same principles can be adapted to other jobs and roles. The idea is to analyze a task and determine how you can do it most easily. Energy saved on routine tasks can then be applied to other activities.

Occupational Rehabilitation

Many of the same energy conservation techniques and principles used for routine daily tasks can be applied to occupational rehabilitation and job training, but the services of an occupational therapist often are needed. For example, many people with chronic lung disorders find it difficult to perform jobs that require extensive use of their arms, because the muscles required for work are often the same ones they need to breathe. Arm-muscle endurance can be improved by using proper breathing techniques and also by specific upper-body exercise conditioning. Occupational therapists also can help people learn how to pace themselves to keep from getting overly tired. Job simplification and the use of assistive devices also may enable a person with asthma and other chronic lung diseases to return to work.

Psychological Support

As noted throughout this book, there is a strong relationship between asthma and emotional factors. The sensation of being unable to breathe, quickly leads to feelings of anxiety and panic, and understandably, people with asthma often will avoid any activity that may provoke an attack. At National Jewish, psychological counseling for both asthma patients and family members is an important aspect of rehabilitation. Frequently, a person with chronic lung disease will be so depressed that he or she is unable to participate in an effective rehabilitation effort. In such instances, diagnosing and treating the depression may have to precede the rehabilitation. Family therapy may be advisable, especially where children are involved. Studies have found that people who have strong psychological and social support systems are more likely to benefit from rehabilitation programs than those who do not.

Making Use of Time

Many asthma patients, especially those who are unable to work or who hold only part-time jobs, find themselves at a loss in regard to filling their time. Susan Barclay recalls that she felt she was turning into a television zombie. "In college, if anyone would have told me that ten years later I would spend most of my time watching General Hospital and the other soaps, I would have told them they were crazy—I had better things to do with my time. But there I was, spending ten or fifteen hours a day gazing at the TV screen."

National Jewish therapists stress the importance of finding satisfying leisure activities that will prevent boredom and offer pleasure and feelings of accomplishment. Many of us feel guilty about relaxation and leisure; however, a good deal depends upon how one defines leisure. To some, working with a volunteer organization is a relaxing leisure-time activity, while for others it is closely akin to a job in that it provides a sense of identification ("I am doing a telephone survey for the American Cancer Society. . . .") and of accomplishment ("We raised enough money through our phone campaign to build a new playground").

"Virtually every community has a long list of resources that people can tap into," a National Jewish worker explained. "We encourage patients, when they feel they have nothing to do, to seek out these resources and find activities that not only fill their time, but also provide companionship, feelings of accomplishment and purpose, and a new interest in life." (The accompanying Table 32 lists possible community resources.)

Table 32
Possible Resources Available in a Community

---

1. City Recreation Department
2. County Recreation Department
3. YMCA
4. YWCA
5. University or college programs
6. Church programs
7. School programs
8. 4H Clubs, Boys' Clubs, Girls' Clubs
9. Parents without Partners Clubs
10. Women's Clubs, Men's Clubs, Senior Citizens' Clubs
11. City Chamber of Commerce (to help locate facilities)
12. Commercial facilities (bowling alleys, skating rinks, etc.)
13. Scouting programs
14. Local theater groups
15. Local library
16. Weight Watchers
17. Alcoholics Anonymous
18. Local stables
19. Welcoming organizations
20. Arts and crafts shops and hobby shops
21. Dance studios

22. Museums
23. Art galleries
24. Local newspapers
25. Community concert association
26. Volunteer service organization
27. Salvation Army
28. Bookstores
29. Garden clubs
30. Yellow pages of telephone book

(From *Pride*, Patient Education Notebook, National Jewish Center for Immunology and Respiratory Medicine.)

A Matter of Outlook

No doubt about it; asthma and other chronic lung disorders can be frustrating and debilitating. Whether a person ends up filled with self-pity and anger, or looks upon asthma as a challenge to be brought under control so he or she can get on with the business of living, is largely a matter of perspective and attitude. Numerous studies have documented that patients who are determined and optimistic do much better than those who feel helpless and out-of-control. Obviously, asthma is not a disease a person can ignore in the hope that it will somehow go away. But for the large majority of patients, it is a disease that can be managed.

In this book, we have presented the basic approach to diagnosis, treatment, and rehabilitation that has been developed at the National Jewish Center for Immunology and Respiratory Medicine in Denver. The tens of thousands of patients who have been helped by this program are testament to its soundness. Ask your doctor if these principles can be applied to your treatment program. National Jewish also will answer questions phoned into its toll-free Lung Line, 1-800-

222-LUNG. There are many things we still do not understand about asthma. Scientists at leading medical research institutions throughout the world, including National Jewish, are working to uncover the underlying biological mechanisms of the disease. Ultimately, understanding asthma will be the key to conquering it. Until then, understanding how to control the disease is the key to living with it.

GLOSSARY

Abscess: A localized collection of pus.

Aerosol: Fine mist containing suspended particles. Inhaled medications are often given in aerosol form.

Air sacs: Common name for alveoli.

Airways: Common name for bronchial tubes, or bronchi.

Allergen: A substance that provokes an allergic reaction.

Allergy: An altered reaction of body tissue to a normally harmless substance (allergen). Common examples include hay fever, hives, etc.

Alveolus (alveoli, plural): Air sac of the lungs. Alveoli are found at the end of bronchial tubes and look like tiny clusters of elastic bubbles. Gas exchange of oxygen and carbon dioxide occurs within alveoli.

Anaphylactic: Rapid onset of an exaggerated allergic response. Can result in collapse, shock, and death.

Angiotensin 2: A chemical formed in lungs that is important in blood-pressure regulation.

Antibiotic: Any of a variety of substances, both natural and manufactured, which slow or prevent the growth of bacteria.

Antibody: A protein substance developed by the body's immune system as a normal protective mechanism.

Anticoagulant: A substance that prevents or delays formation of blood clots.

Antigen: A substance that stimulates the formation of antibodies.

Antihistamine: Substance that reduces effects of histamines in treatment of allergies.

Arterial blood gas: A blood test that tells how much oxygen and carbon dioxide are present in the bloodstream.

Atelectasis: A collapsed or airless condition of the lung. May be caused by obstruction, foreign bodies, mucus plugs, or excessive secretions.

Basophils: White blood cells that carry specific antibodies on their surface and secrete substances that produce an allergic reaction.

Belly breathing: Breathing maneuver that uses diaphragm as major muscle in inhalation.

Beta-2 agonists: Bronchodilating drugs that act on receptors to relax bronchial muscles. Used to treat and prevent asthma attacks.

Beta blockers: Drugs that may cause bronchial constriction as a negative side effect. Commonly used for heart disorders and high blood pressure; usually contraindicated for asthmatics.

Bone demineralization: Loss of normal mineral composition of bones; common complication of long-term steroid therapy.

Bronchial tubes: Common name for bronchus (singular) or bronchi (plural). Passageways for air moving to and from the lungs. Bronchial tubes branch into smaller and smaller passageways, ending in alveoli.

Bronchioles: Small airways branching off the bronchi.

Bronchiectasis: Abnormal dilation of bronchus or bronchi which is associated with a large amount of mucus secretion and/or pus.

Bronchitis: Inflammation of the bronchial tubes.

Bronchodilator: Medication used to open up or dilate bronchial tubes. Prescribed both as a preventive and treatment for asthma.

Bronchogram: X ray using a radio-opaque material to visualize the bronchial tree.

Bronchoscope: Flexible tube with fiberoptic viewing devices used to examine respiratory tree.

Bronchoscopy: Examination of the bronchi using an instrument called a bronchoscope.

Bronchospasm: Constriction of air passages caused by bronchial muscle contraction.

Carbon dioxide: A colorless, harmless gas, produced as normal part of metabolism. Removed from the body via the lungs in exhaled air.

Carbon monoxide: A dangerous gas found in automobile exhaust and cigarette smoke.

Chronic obstructive pulmonary disease (COPD): Disease process that causes decreased ability of lungs to function. Common examples include emphysema, chronic bronchitis, or bronchiectasis.

Cilia: Tiny hairlike structures that have a wavelike motion. Those located in air passageways move mucus, pus, dust, and other debris out of the lungs into the windpipe where it can be coughed up. Cigarette smoking and certain diseases, such as cystic fibrosis, can damage the lung's cilia.

Constriction: Narrowing or tightening of an opening.

Corticosteroids: Adrenal hormones used to treat asthma and a wide variety of other diseases. Reduce inflammation in bronchial passages. Common examples are prednisone, cortisone, and beclomethasone.

Cor pulmonale: Failure of right side of heart due to lung disorders.

Cough syncope: Coughing so hard that it results in fainting.

Cromolyn sodium: Medication that prevents bronchospasm; used prophylactically in asthma.

Cyanosis: Slightly bluish or grayish color of skin due to lack of oxygen.

Diaphragm: Large, dome-shaped muscle that separates chest from abdomen. It is major breathing muscle.

Diaphragmatic training: Exercises to increase use of diaphragm in breathing.

Dilation: Expanding or spreading apart of an opening.

Dyspnea: Air hunger resulting in labored or difficult breathing.

Ear oximeter: A device to measure amount of oxygen in bloodstream.

Edema: Excessive accumulation of fluid in body tissues, causing swelling and weight gain.

Elimination diet: A diet initially restricted to a few normally nonallergenic foods; followed by testing of suspected individual foods, one at a time, and observing for signs of allergic reaction.

Emphysema: A chronic lung disease in which alveoli lose their elasticity and become distended, with eventual destruction of walls.

Epiglottis: A lid-like structure at the top of the larynx that closes during swallowing to prevent food and water from entering the trachea.

Epinephrine: Adrenalin; used in emergency treatment of acute bronchospasm and anaphylaxis.

Esophagus: Muscular tube through which food travels from mouth to stomach.

Exhale: Breathe out.

Extrinsic asthma: Asthma triggered by exposure to an allergen.

FEV$_1$: Forced expiratory volume in one second; amount of air expelled in one second after a big breath.

FEV: Forced vital capacity; amount of air that can be expelled after a big breath.

Gas exchange: Process in which oxygen is picked up by the blood as it passes through the lungs, and carbon dioxide is removed from the blood.

Generic: General name for drugs available for common use that are not protected by a brand name.

Goblet cell: A type of secretory cell found in the lining of the respiratory tract and which is responsible for secreting mucus.

Hay fever: Popular term for allergic disease of the mucous passages of nose and upper passages.

Hemoptysis: Spitting or coughing up of blood.

Histamine: A chemical substance normally present in the body, which is released when tissues are injured.

Hyperreactive airways: Airways that become tight, twitchy, or narrowed when exposed to normally harmless substances. Also called hyperactive, hypersensitive.

Hyperventilation: Increased inspiration and expiration as a result of deeper and/or faster breathing. Can cause marked anxiety, dizziness, fainting, and other symptoms.

Hypoventilation: Reduced rate and depth of respiration.

Hypoxia: Lack of adequate oxygen in body tissues.

Immune system: Defense mechanisms of the body that protect against invasion of disease and foreign substances.

Immunoglobin E (IgE): An antibody that normally protects body from foreign organisms. In extrinsic asthma, an excess of IgE causes release of substances that produce an allergic reaction.

Immunotherapy: Allergy shots. Chronic administration of small amounts of an allergen to desensitize the body to it.

Inflammation: Tissue reaction to injury, irritation, and/or infection. Often results in swelling, tenderness, and redness of injured tissue.

Inhalation therapy: Administration of drugs, water, vapors, and/or gases to the lungs by breathing in. Drugs usually are misted by using an aerosol or spray apparatus.

Inhale: To breath in.

Interstitial lung disease: An inflammatory lung disease that affects the spaces between the cells, resulting in stiffness of lung tissue and making inhalation difficult.

Intrinsic asthma: Asthma associated with other respiratory conditions, such as sinusitis or bronchitis.

Intravenous infusion: Injection of a drug or solution into a vein. Commonly called IV.

IPPB: Intermittent positive pressure breathing; a machine used to assist in breathing.

Larynx: Voice box.

Lobectomy: Surgical removal of a lobe from the lung.

Lobes: Sections of the lungs. The right lung is divided into three lobes; the left into two.

Mast cell: A cell found in connective tissue, including that of the bronchial tubes. Contains histamine and other substances that are instrumental in an allergic reaction.

Medulla: A section of the lower brain containing centers that control respiration, swallowing, coughing, and other reflex functions.

Metabolism: The chemical changes in living cells by which energy is provided for body functioning.

Metered-dose inhaler: Device used to deliver asthma medication in aerosol form. Also called a whiffer.

Mixed asthma: A combination of extrinsic and intrinsic asthma.

Muscle atrophy: A wasting away or shrinking of muscle tissue.

Muscle myopathy: A muscle disease or abnormality.

Mucus: Clear, slippery fluid secreted by mucous membranes lining the bronchial tubes. Commonly called phlegm or sputum.

Nebulizer: An atomizer or sprayer that creates a fine mist or spray, which can be inhaled into lungs.

Orthopnea: Respiratory disorder in which there is discomfort in breathing while lying down.

Paroxysmal: A sudden, periodic attack or recurrence of symptoms of a disease.

Peak-flow meter: Portable device designed for use by a patient to measure air flow as it is expelled from the lungs.

Pleura: Serous membrane or covering of the lungs; attached to walls of the chest cavity and diaphragm.

Pleurisy: Inflammation or irritation of pleura.

Pneumonectomy: Surgical removal of a lung.

Pneumonia: Inflammation of lungs, usually caused by bacteria or viruses; also may be caused by chemical irritants and allergies.

Postural drainage: Drainage of secretions from bronchi by placing patient's head lower than chest or lungs; often accompanied by coughing and clapping, or by tapping chest.

Pulmonary function tests: Breathing tests to determine how well lungs are functioning.

Rales: Abnormal sound heard in lungs produced by air passing through a narrowed passage or one containing moisture.

Residual air: Air remaining in lungs after strongest possible forced expiration.

ROAD: Reversible obstructive airway disease; technical term for asthma.

Sinus: Space within skull that communicates with the air passages by way of throat or nose.

Sinusitis: Infection in the sinus.

Skin test: Injection of a fluid substance under the skin to test for reaction or sensitivity to a substance.

Spasm: A sudden tightening or constriction.

Spirometer: A device used in testing lung function.

Spirometry: Lung function tests.

Sputum: Fluid substance brought up when coughing or clearing throat.

Steroids: A term embracing naturally occurring chemicals akin to cholesterol and including sex and adrenal cortical hormones. (See corticosteroids.)

Theophylline: Asthma drugs in xanthine family. Chemically related to caffeine; work by relaxing bronchial passages and stimulating central nervous system.

Trachea: Windpipe.

Tracheitis: Inflammation of the trachea.

Triggers: Conditions or substances that initiate asthma attacks.

Wheeze: A whistling or sighing sound caused by narrowing of the respiratory passage. Usually accompanied by difficult breathing; a common symptom of asthma.

INDEX